Understand Your

DIABETES

and Live a Healthy Life

Publisher: Caroline Bélisle
Project Manager: Chantal Benhamron
Art Director: Marie-Josée Forest
Desktop Designers: Jocelyne Demers, Dino Peressini
Business Manager: Geneviève Cimon
Manager, Book Division: Louis Audet

Cover page image: Lina Arvidsson/Plainpicture/Maskot
Inside page images: iStockphoto

Rogers Publishing Limited, HealthCare Group
1200 McGill College avenue, Suite 800
Montréal (Québec) H3B 4G7
514 845-5141

Understand Your Diabetes and Live a Healthy Life
ISBN 978-2-922260-30-4
Legal Deposit: 3rd quarter 2013
Bibliothèque et Archives nationales du Québec 2013
Library and Archives Canada 2013

The publication of this book was made possible thanks to
an unrestricted educational grant from Sanofi.

SANOFI

Printing: Transcontinental Interglobe, Beauceville, Canada

METABOLIC MEDICINE DAY-CARE CENTRE – CHUM - HÔTEL-DIEU, MONTREAL

Understand Your
DIABETES
and Live a Healthy Life

In collaboration with Dr. Robert G Josse
Division of Endocrinology and Metabolism, St. Michael's Hospital,
Professor of Medicine, University of Toronto

RECOMMENDED BY

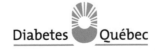

Diabetes Québec

NEW REVISED AND EXPANDED EDITION

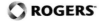
ROGERS

Preface

Diabetes is a malevolent stranger. Uninvited, it creeps into your daily life, disrupting your existence, both physically and psychologically. Suddenly, every aspect of your life and work is affected by this unwelcome guest, who has moved in and set up headquarters in your body.

To some people, the disease might seem unremarkable or harmless. And actually, this is not surprising: why should it be taken seriously, when it causes no symptoms, no pain, no bleeding – in short, no visible physical signs at all? But this is precisely how diabetes operates. Deceptively harmless and innocent at first, it hides its true intentions as it quietly works towards its destructive goal. But the situation is not desperate, on the contrary. There are ways to prevent it from achieving its harmful objectives.

Reading this book is an excellent first step. The information it provides will help you understand your adversary better and give you the tools you need to control it. This process will involve numerous changes, many that might seem minor but that in fact hold the key to the successful management of your diabetes.

Your new lifestyle will also require a whole new language, one that might seem intimidating at first. Blood glucose, hypoglycemia, hyperglycemia, carbohydrates, insulin… the list goes on, and it is easy to lose your bearings. There are also a number of myths about diabetes, many of them durable and superficially more appealing or interesting than reality. The Internet is not always the best place to debunk them. You need solid, reliable sources to help you find your way through the maze.

This book is one of those sources. It will guide you through the daily reality of living with and managing diabetes. Use it as you would a GPS – rely on it when you don't know where to go, when the path seems winding and strewn with traps. Read it from cover to cover, and keep it on hand as a reference tool that to help you understand your diabetes, manage it successfully, and above all, live a healthy life.

Serge Langlois
President-Director General
Diabetes Québec

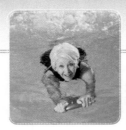
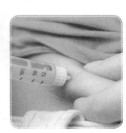
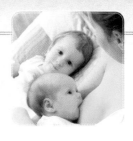

Foreword

Here is another edition of *Understand Your Diabetes and Live a Healthy Life*.

Diabetes has a long history. The ancient Greeks used the term dia-baino, which means "to pass through," to describe people who urinated as soon as they took a drink. Thankfully, our understanding of diabetes, its causes, diagnosis, complications, treatment and prevention has never stopped evolving. It is now possible to prevent or delay the onset of type 2 diabetes by adopting a healthy lifestyle and taking certain medications.

It is very important for people with diabetes or at risk of developing the disease to be aware of new discoveries and approaches. This type of knowledge can help them change their lifestyles and make it easier to take control of this chronic disease, which is rapidly increasing in occurrence.

We hope that this book will be a valuable source of information for the population in general. More specifically, we hope that it can motivate people with diabetes to achieve a better understanding of themselves and their relationship to the disease and learn how to improve their treatment so that they can get the most out of life.

CHUM–Hotel-Dieu Metabolic Medicine Day-care Centre

List of Authors

This book has been re-edited by the multidisciplinary team of the Centre hospitalier de l'Universite de Montreal, Hotel-Dieu, namely:

- Sophie Bernard, endocrinologist
- Chantal Cormier, nurse
- Françoise Desrochers, nurse clinician
- Lyne Gauthier, pharmacist
- Michelle Messier, dietitian
- Catherine Noulard, dietitian
- Thérèse Surprenant, dietitian
- Cynthia Turcotte, psychologist
- Lucretia Virlan, nurse

We would also like to acknowledge the work done by the authors who contributed to previous editions:

- Nathalie Beaulieu, dietitian
- Jean-Louis Chiasson, endocrinologist
- Julie Demers, pharmacist
- Micheline Fecteau-Côté, dietitian
- Sylvie Fournier, pharmacist
- Christiane Gobeil, dietitian
- Nicole Hamel, pharmacist
- Lise Lussier, psychologist
- Hortensia Mircescu, endocrinologist
- Caroline Rivest, pharmacist
- Charles Tourigny, psychologist
- Danièle Tremblay, psychologist
- Francis Viguié, psychologist

Acknowledgments

We would like to thank the members of the Division of Endocrinology-Metabolism and Nutrition of the CHUM-Hotel-Dieu for their contribution, and in particular Dr. Ariane Godbout, Dr. Jean-Marie Ékoé and Dr. Rémi Rabasa-Lhoret. We are also grateful to Ms. Susanne Bordeleau for her work as coordinator.

We would also like to express our gratitude to the following health professionals for their revisions, comments, and suggestions:

- Marc Aras, Director of Communications, Diabetes Québec
- Andrée Gagné, dietician, Diabetes Québec
- Julie St-Jean, dietician, Diabetes Québec
- Louise Tremblay, nurse and M.Ed., Diabetes Quebec

Objectives of This Book

This book has the following objectives:

General objective
To help people with diabetes achieve optimal control of their health so that they may improve their well-being and reduce the risk of developing complications of diabetes.

Specific objectives
To provide tools to people with diabetes to help them improve their habits, maintain normal blood glucose levels, and enable them to:
- acquire general knowledge about diabetes;
- adapt their diet to their diabetes and their various activities;
- take into account the effects of stress and physical exercise on the management of their disease;
- recognize the complications caused by poorly controlled blood glucose levels;
- take effective steps when complications do occur;
- recognize situations that require emergency intervention;
- understand the treatments (such as drugs and insulin) that are used to treat diabetes and its complications;
- understand the adjustments necessary in special situations (for example, while exercising or on trips);
- understand the importance of good foot care and general hygiene;
- correctly operate blood glucose measurement and insulin delivery devices;
- use community resources, when needed;
- adopt a positive attitude and management strategies to take better control of their health.

Table of Contents

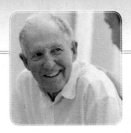

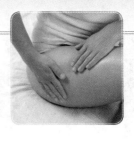

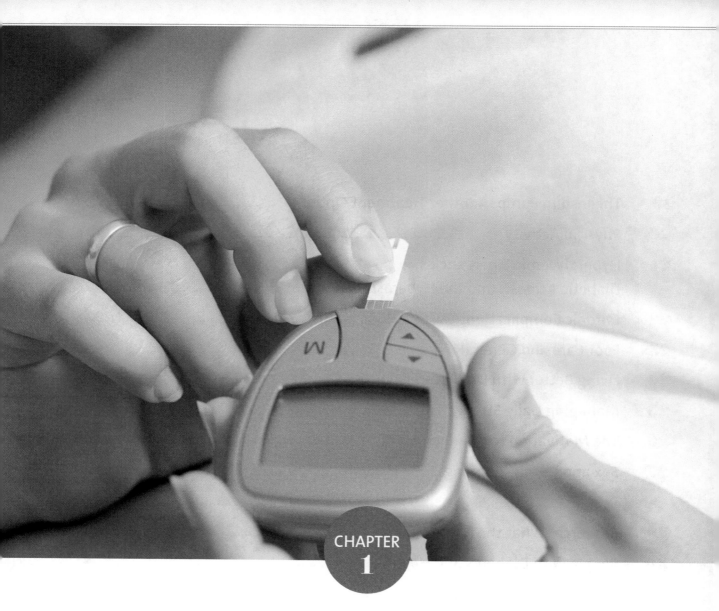

General Information about Diabetes

1

What is diabetes?

Diabetes is a disease characterized by a lack of insulin and/or impaired insulin action, which causes an **elevation of blood glucose** (blood sugar) to above normal levels.

2

How many Canadians have diabetes?

About 2.4 million Canadians (6.8% of the population) had diabetes in 2009. It is anticipated that the number of cases will be 3.7 million by 2019, making diabetes the **disease of the 21st century**. Diabetes engenders increasingly significant societal costs and is a growing problem that must be battled on all fronts.

3

What are the criteria for a diagnosis of diabetes?

A diabetes diagnosis is based on results of laboratory tests performed on venous blood indicating:

- **fasting blood glucose** equal to or above 7.0 mmol/L;
- **random blood glucose** equal to or above 11.1 mmol/L;
- **oral glucose tolerance test (OGTT)**, with a blood glucose level equal to or above 11.1 mmol/L two hours after the consumption of 75 g of glucose;

- **glycated hemoglobin (A1C)** equal to or greater than 6.5%.

If there are no symptoms, a medical diagnosis of diabetes requires that an abnormal result on one of these tests be confirmed by repeating one of the tests on a different day.

4

What is normal blood glucose?

Blood glucose is considered normal when it is below **6.1 mmol/L before meals, and below 7.8 mmol/L two hours after drinking a beverage containing 75 g of glucose.**

5

What are the target blood glucose levels in diabetes treatment?

The **target glucose levels** for most people with diabetes should be between 4 mmol/L and 7 mmol/L before meals, and between 5 mmol/L and 10 mmol/L two hours after meals. Target glucose levels after meals should be individualized to the patient. If diabetes control is not optimal (A1C greater than 7%), levels after meals should be between 5 mmol/L and 8 mmol/L.

Why is a normal or target blood glucose level important?

The closer blood glucose is to normal, the more a person with diabetes will:

- feel fit, and
- lower the risk of long-term complications associated with diabetes.

Why does a person with diabetes have higher blood glucose levels?

Blood glucose rises because of a **lack of insulin**, which can be caused by reduced insulin secretion, decreased insulin action, or a combination of the two. When there is **insufficient insulin** or insulin action to enable glucose to enter the cells, glucose levels in the blood increase. This is called **hyperglycemia**.

What is insulin?

Insulin is a hormone produced by the **pancreas**, an organ located in the abdomen, behind the stomach.

Insulin is like a **key that opens the door to let glucose enter the cells**, thus ensuring that glucose in the blood remains within normal range.

How does the body use glucose?

Much as gasoline is a necessary fuel for cars, glucose is a vital **energy source** for the body's cells.

Where does the excess glucose in the blood of a person with diabetes come from?

Excess glucose in the blood comes from two sources:

- foods containing **carbohydrates in meals and snacks**;
- the **liver**, when its glucose production is not properly regulated.

What are the characteristics of type 1 diabetes?

Typically, type 1 diabetes is characterized by the following:

- **a total lack of insulin**;
- the appearance of the disease **around puberty** or in early adulthood (usually **before age 40**)
- weight loss;
- the need for treatment with insulin injections.

What are the characteristics of type 2 diabetes?

Typically, type 2 diabetes is characterized by the following:

- **insulin resistance**, where the insulin produced becomes less effective;
- **insufficient insulin production**;
- appearance of the disease **after age 40** (although in certain populations at risk, it is becoming increasingly frequent in younger people);
- **excess weight**;
- **family history**;
- treatment through lifestyle modification (diet, increased physical activity) **alone** or in combination with **oral antidiabetic drugs. In some cases, insulin injections are necessary.**

Are some people predisposed to diabetes?

Yes. Susceptibility to diabetes is genetically inherited.

Are there factors that can trigger diabetes in people who are predisposed?

Yes, there are a number of external (i.e. non genetic) factors that can trigger the disease in those with a predisposition. Certain viral infections, for example, can precipitate type 1 diabetes in people who are predisposed. As for type 2 diabetes, two major factors play roles in its development: excess weight and lack of physical activity. Physical or physiological stress such as heart attacks, strokes, or infections can also trigger the development of diabetes, especially type 2, in predisposed individuals. It can also be brought on by psychological stressors such as the loss of a loved one. Certain drugs – for example, high doses of cortisone or antipsychotics – can also be triggers.

Can some diseases cause diabetes?

Yes, some diseases can cause diabetes. Cystic fibrosis and pancreatitis (inflammation of the pancreas) can destroy the pancreas, bringing on the disease. Other conditions such as gestational diabetes, polycystic ovary syndrome, schizophrenia and certain types of muscular dystrophy also increase the risk of developing type 2 diabetes.

Are there tests to identify people who are predisposed to developing type 2 diabetes?

There are tests to identify people with an elevated risk of developing the disease. A fasting blood glucose level above 6 mmol/L but below 7 mmol/L is considered **an abnormal fasting blood glucose level**, and is known as **impaired fasting blood glucose (IFG)**. In addition, blood glucose anywhere between 7.8 mmol/L and 11.0 mmol/L two hours after drinking a beverage containing 75 g of glucose can indicate **impaired glucose tolerance (IGT)**. Finally, A1C between 6.0% and 6.4% is considered abnormal.

These three states — impaired fasting blood glucose, impaired glucose tolerance, and A1C between 6.0% and 6.4% — are considered prediabetic and indicate an elevated risk of developing the disease.

Reactive hypoglycemia (a drop below normal blood glucose levels, usually three to four hours after a meal containing carbohydrates) is sometimes the first sign of type 2 diabetes.

Individuals with a fasting blood glucose between 5.6 mmol/L and 6.0 mmol/L and/or A1C between 5.5% and 5.9% are at risk of prediabetes and should be screened more often than individuals with fasting blood glucose below 5.6 mmol/L and A1C below 5.5%.

Is it possible to prevent or slow down the development of diabetes in prediabetic people?

Yes. It has been shown that weight loss and physical activity can decrease the risk of developing type 2 diabetes by over 50% in people who are glucose intolerant. Certain medications (metformin, acarbose) have also been shown to be effective, decreasing the risk of developing diabetes in subjects with impaired glucose tolerance by over 30%.

How can a person with diabetes achieve and maintain target or normal blood glucose?

People have to take responsibility of the disease to be able to control it. The following guidelines can help:

- **acknowledge and accept** the condition;
- **eat** healthy food;
- **lose weight**, if necessary;
- be **physically active**;
- measure **blood glucose** regularly;
- take antidiabetic **drugs** and/or insulin as prescribed;
- learn to **manage** stress;
- stay well **informed** about diabetes.

As a person with diabetes, you are the one
best equipped to manage it— with the help and
support of your doctor and other
health care professionals, of course.

———

Diabetes is a chronic disease. It cannot be cured,
but it can be controlled.

———

You have done nothing to bring on your diabetes,
and there is no reason to feel guilty.

———

The closer you keep your blood glucose to normal,
the better you will feel.

———

The more you learn about your diabetes, the more
you will be able to take responsibility for it.

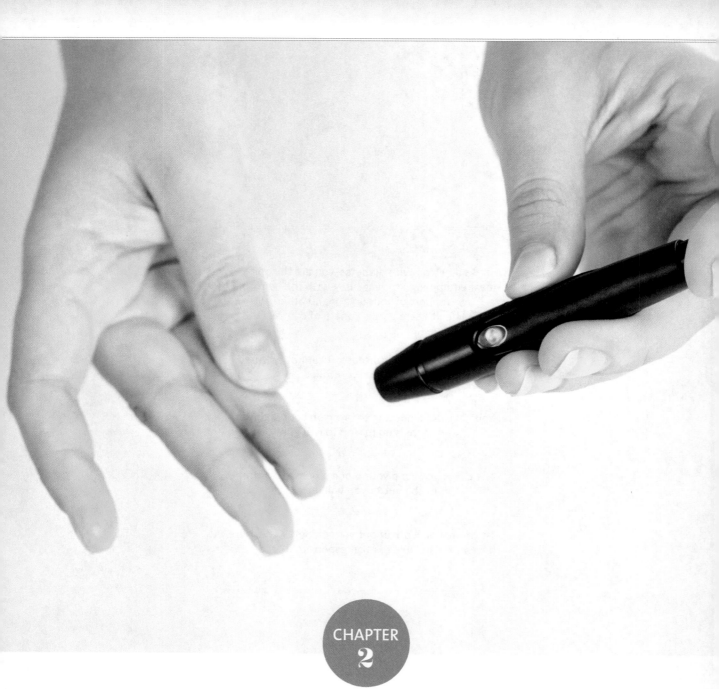

Hyperglycemia

What is hyperglycemia?

Hyperglycemia occurs when **blood glucose rises above target levels**, that is, above 7 mmol/L before meals and above 10 mmol/L two hours after the beginning of a meal.

How do people with diabetes develop hyperglycemia?

People with diabetes develop hyperglycemia when there is an **insufficient amount of insulin in the blood to handle the amount of glucose being released into the bloodstream.**

What are the symptoms of hyperglycemia?

When blood glucose rises above a certain threshold, the following symptoms can appear:

- dry **mouth**;
- intense **thirst**;
- **increase in the volume of urine and the frequency of urination**;
- excessive **hunger**;
- involuntary **weight loss**.

Hyperglycemia can also cause the following symptoms:

- **blurred vision**;
- **infections**, especially of the genital organs and bladder;
- **sores or ulcers** that heal very slowly;
- **fatigue**;
- **drowsiness**;
- **irritability**.

What are the main causes of hyperglycemia?

The main causes of hyperglycemia are:

- over-consumption of **foods** containing carbohydrates;
- **decreased physical activity**;
- **insufficient insulin or medications** (e.g., incorrect dosage of antidiabetic drugs and/or insulin);
- **infection**;
- poorly managed **stress**;
- taking certain **medications** (e.g., cortisone);
- **uncorrected nocturnal hypoglycemia** followed by a hyperglycemic rebound in the morning.

What should a person with diabetes do if hyperglycemia is suspected?

If you suspect you have hyperglycemia, measure your blood glucose.

If hyperglycemia is confirmed, the following steps are necessary:

1 People with type 1 diabetes must check for ketone bodies if blood glucose is higher than 14 mmol/L. Reagent strips (Chemstrip® uG/K, Keto-Diastix®, Ketostix®) can measure the level of ketone bodies in the urine, and a meter (such as NovaMax® Plus™, Precision Xtra®) is used to measure the level of ketone bodies in a blood sample taken from the fingertip.

2 Drink plenty of water to avoid dehydration (250 mL of water per hour, unless contraindicated).

3 Identify the cause of the hyperglycemia.

4 Correct the cause if possible.

5 Continue eating (including carbohydrates) and follow the prescribed treatment (oral antidiabetic drugs or insulin).

6 Call the doctor if the situation does not correct itself.

7 Call the doctor or go to the emergency room in the following situations:

Blood glucose levels:

- If you have type 1 diabetes and your blood glucose rises above 20 mmol/L with moderate to high levels of ketone bodies, with or without vomiting.

- if you have type 2 diabetes and your blood glucose rises above 30 mmol/L, or it is impossible to retain liquids taken orally because of nausea and vomiting.

Ketone bodies:

There are different methods to measure ketone bodies in urine or blood.

- If the level of ketone bodies in your urine is moderate (4 mmol/L) to high (16 mmol/L), using Ketostix®;

- If using another product (e.g., Chemstrip® uG/K or Keto-Diastix®), refer to the instructions on how to read the results and store the strips;

- If the level of ketone bodies in blood taken from the fingertip using the Precision Xtra® reader is above 3 mmol/L. If using the NovaMax® Plus™ reader, refer to the manufacturer's instructions.

What are the long-term complications of hyperglycemia?

In the long term, hyperglycemia can cause complications affecting the eyes, kidneys, nerves, heart, and blood vessels.[1]

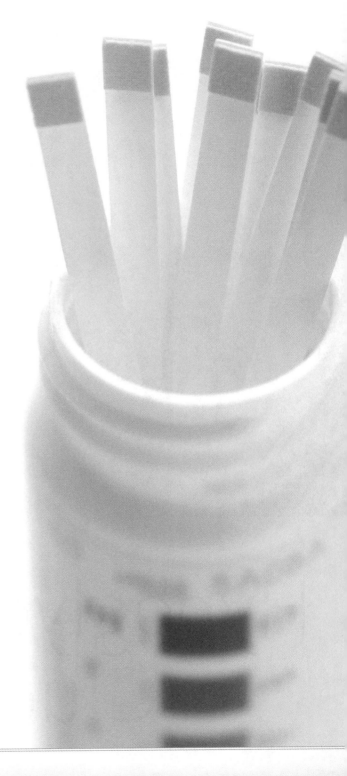

1 Canadian Diabetes Association Clinical Practice Guidelines Expert Committee. Canadian Diabetes Association, 2013 Clinical Practice Guidelines for the Prevention and Management of Diabetes in Canada. *Can. J. Diabetes 2013*; 37 (suppl. 1):S1-S212.

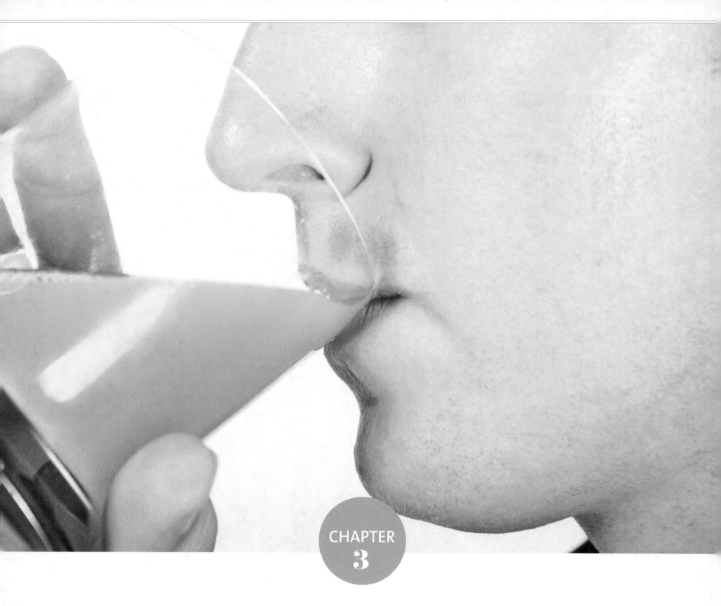

Hypoglycemia and Glucagon

What is hypoglycemia?

Hypoglycemia occurs when blood glucose levels drop below normal (below 4 mmol/L).

Why do people with diabetes develop hypoglycemia?

People with diabetes can develop hypoglycemia when there is too much insulin in the blood in relation to the amount of glucose entering the circulation.

Who is susceptible to hypoglycemia?

People who inject insulin or who take medications that stimulate the pancreas to produce more insulin can develop hypoglycemia. These medications include chlorpropamide (Apo®-Chlorpropamide), tolbutamide (Apo®-Tolbutamide), glyburide (Diaßeta®, Euglucon®), gliclazide (Diamicron® and Diamicron® MR), glimepiride (Amaryl®), repaglinide (GlucoNorm®) and nateglinide (Starlix®).

What are the symptoms of hypoglycemia?

The body has two types of warning systems. The first causes rapid onset symptoms, brought on by the secretion of adrenalin.

When hypoglycemia develops rapidly, it can cause the following symptoms:

- tremors or shakes;
- palpitations;
- sweating;
- anxiety;
- acute hunger;
- pallor;
- nausea;
- nightmares and restless sleep, if the hypoglycemia occurs during sleep;
- waking with a headache and rebound hyperglycemia in the morning following uncorrected nocturnal hypoglycemia during the night before.

The second warning system creates generally less perceptible symptoms with slower onset. These symptoms are caused by a shortage of glucose being carried to the brain.

When hypoglycemia occurs slowly, the symptoms are more subtle:
- numbness or tingling around the mouth;
- yawning;
- fatigue or weakness;
- the urge to sleep;
- mood swings;
- difficulty concentrating;
- dizziness;
- blurred vision;
- unsteady gait, poor coordination;
- difficulty pronouncing words;
- confusion;
- aggressiveness.

Does hypoglycemia always cause these symptoms?

No. The symptoms of hypoglycemia vary from person to person and can change over time. Sometimes hypoglycemia is asymptomatic, especially if blood glucose drops slowly or the person has had diabetes for many years. The more frequent the hypoglycemia, the more likely it is that warning symptoms will appear late and the correction of the problem delayed.

What are the causes of hypoglycemia?

The most common causes of hypoglycemia can be broken down into three categories:

Food:
- skipping a snack or a meal;
- delaying a meal;
- insufficient consumption of foods containing carbohydrates;
- an error in measuring the carbohydrate content of food;
- inability to retain food (vomiting, diarrhea);
- drinking alcohol (this can lead to hypoglycemia as long as 24 hours after consumption);
- fasting while taking antidiabetic medications;
- gastroparesis (delayed emptying of the contents of the stomach).

Physical activity:
- physical activity without adjusting the intake of food or medication.

Antidiabetic drugs:
- incorrect (excessive) dosage of antidiabetic drugs or insulin;
- overcorrection of high blood glucose by injecting too much insulin;
- failure to adjust to a lower dosage, despite glucose levels frequently below 4 mmol/L;
- improper timing of antidiabetic drug doses.

What are the different degrees of hypoglycemia?

Mild:

- physical symptoms (trembling, palpitations, sweating, hunger, nausea);
- self-treatment is possible.

Moderate:

- physical and neurological symptoms (headache, changes in vision, dizziness, irritability);
- self-treatment for hypoglycemia is possible.

Severe:

- self-treatment is not possible; help from another person is required;
- possible loss of consciousness.

What should people with diabetes do if mild or moderate hypoglycemia is suspected?

If you suspect the onset of hypoglycemia, do not go to sleep without treating the hypoglycemia, assuming that your blood glucose level will correct itself.

Instead, do the following:

- measure your blood glucose;
- eat food with 15 g of rapidly absorbed carbohydrates. Glucose or sucrose (sugar) in pill or liquid form is the best option;
- wait 15 minutes;
- measure your blood glucose again; if hypoglycemia is still present, eat an additional 15 g of carbohydrates.

Examples of foods providing approximately 15 g of carbohydrates:

1st choice (quickest absorption)

- 4 tables of Dex4®
  (1 tablet = 4 g of carbohydrates)
- 59 mL of Dex4® liquid
  (1 bottle = 16 g of carbohydrates)
- 5 tablets of Dextro®
  (1 tablet = 3 g of carbohydrates)
- 7 tablets of Glucosol®
  (1 tablet = 2.25 g of carbohydrates)
- 15 mL (3 tsp or 3 packets) of sugar dissolved in water
- 15 mL (3 tsp) of maple or corn syrup

2nd choice (slower absorption)

- 125 mL to 175 mL (½ to ¾ cup) of regular (not diet) soft drink (pop) or fruit beverage
- 125 mL to 175 mL (½ to ¾ cup) of fruit juice without added sugar
- 1 dried fruit bar (for example, "Fruit To Go")
- 1 small apple or ½ banana or 2 kiwis or 2 dates, etc.
- 1 tube Dex4® gel
  (1 tube = 17 g of carbohydrates)

If the hypoglycemia is corrected but the next meal is over an hour away, have a snack containing 15 g of carbohydrates and a protein source (e.g., 300 mL of milk or a piece of fruit with cheese).

Note: Do not over-treat hypoglycemia, as this can cause rebound hyperglycemia and weight gain.

What should be done if the person with diabetes suspects severe hypoglycemia?

If the person with diabetes is unable to administer his or her own treatment and needs help from someone else:

- measure his or her blood glucose level, if possible;
- give the person food containing 20 g of rapidly absorbed carbohydrates;
- if needed, repeat after 15 minutes with 15 g of carbohydrates if the person is unable to do it or if blood glucose remains lower than 4 mmol/L.

Examples of quickly absorbed foods containing 20 g of carbohydrates:

1st choice (quickest absorption)
- 5 tablets of Dex4®
  (1 tablet = 4 g of carbohydrates)
- 7 tablets of Dextro®
  (1 tablet = 3 g of carbohydrates)
- 9 tablets of Glucosol®
  (1 tablet = 2.25 g of carbohydrates)

- 20 mL (4 tsp) or 4 packets of sugar dissolved in water

2nd choice (slower absorption)
- 175 mL (¾ cup) of regular soft drink (not diet) or fruit beverage
- 1 tube Insta-Glucose
  (1 tube = 24 g of carbohydrates)

Why is it important to treat hypoglycemia immediately?

Hypoglycemia must be treated immediately because if left uncorrected, it can lead to loss of consciousness, coma, and sometimes convulsions. So called "minor hypoglycemia" should not be neglected as it can get worse and become more and seriously symptomatic.

Does uncorrected hypoglycemia always lead to coma?

No, uncorrected hypoglycemia does not necessarily lead to coma. The body attempts to defend itself from hypoglycemia by secreting hormones such as glucagon and adrenalin, which can elevate blood glucose and correct hypoglycemia. If there is too much insulin in the blood, however, these efforts might not be sufficient to correct hypoglycemia and prevent coma.

How can hypoglycemia be avoided?

The following precautions are usually effective ways of avoiding hypoglycemia:

- Measure blood glucose regularly.
- Keep regular meal times and include foods containing carbohydrates.
- Check blood glucose before beginning any physical activity and eat carbohydrates as needed (*see chapter 20 on Physical Activity, page 184*);
- Avoid drinking alcohol on an empty stomach.
- If nocturnal hypoglycemia is suspected, check blood glucose around 2 a.m.
- Take antidiabetic drugs as prescribed, following the recommended dosage and timetable.

Note: Measuring blood sugar regularly may not be appropriate for all patients with type 2 diabetes, but should be done in those on antidiabetic drugs that cause hypoglycemia or of course those on insulin.

People with type 1 diabetes are advised to check blood glucose around 2 a.m. periodically. If blood glucose is below 7 mmol/L at bedtime, a snack with at least 15 g of carbohydrates and a protein source is also recommended before turning in for the night.

What safety measures should be taken by people with diabetes who are at risk for hypoglycemia?

People with diabetes at risk for hypoglycemia must:

- always keep at least two 15 g servings of carbohydrates within reach;
- wear a diabetic ID bracelet or pendant;
- inform family, friends and colleagues that they have diabetes and tell them about the symptoms of hypoglycemia and the way to deal with it;
- if they take insulin, always have glucagon within reach at home, at work or when travelling. A friend or relative must learn how to inject the glucagon in the event of a hypoglycemic coma.

What should be done if a person with diabetes has fallen into a hypoglycemic coma?

If a person with diabetes is unconscious or in a hypoglycemic coma, another person must immediately:

- inject him or her with glucagon, if available; if not,
- dial 911 for an ambulance.

Never try to feed sugary foods to an unconscious person because there is a risk that the food will be inhaled into the bronchial tubes instead of swallowed into the stomach

What does glucagon do?

Glucagon is a hormone produced by the pancreas that elevates blood glucose. In the event of a hypoglycemic coma, another person must inject glucagon to correct glucose levels.

There are two types of first-aid equipment for this type of emergency: glucagon for injection and the GlucaGen® Hypokit. They can be stored at room temperature. Check the expiry date periodically.

Here are the steps to follow in the event of a hypoglycemic coma:

- Lay the person on his or her side (glucagon can occasionally cause nausea and vomiting).
- Remove the plastic cap from the bottle of glucagon.
- Remove the needle sheath and inject the entire contents of the syringe into the bottle of glucagon. Do not remove the plastic stop ring from the syringe. Remove the syringe from the bottle.
- Gently shake the bottle until the glucagon powder is completely dissolved in the solvent.
- Draw up all of the solution from the vial using the same syringe.
- Inject the contents of the syringe (1 mg) subcutaneously (under the skin) or intramuscularly. The person should wake up within 15 minutes. There is no risk of overdose. A doctor may recommend a half dose for children who weigh less than 20 kg (44 pounds).

- Give the person some food as soon as he or she is awake and able to swallow. Provide a meal or a normal snack according to the usual schedule.
- If the meal is more than an hour away, provide a snack containing 45 g of carbohydrates and some protein (e.g., 300 mL of milk or fruit with cheese).
- Inform the person's doctor of the incident so that treatment can be evaluated and possibly adjusted. A visit to the emergency room may still be necessary to follow up on the correction of the hypoglycemia.

A person with diabetes who does not regain consciousness within 15 or 20 minutes after the glucagon is administered should be taken to the emergency room immediately.

Are there any recommendations for people with diabetes who live alone and are at risk of developing nocturnal hypoglycemia?

People with diabetes who live alone may be apprehensive about nocturnal hypoglycemia. They should remember, however, that hypoglycemia rarely persists for extended periods of time. In a crisis situation, the body reacts by increasing blood glucose with sugar stored in the liver. Nevertheless, hypoglycemia is stressful, so in addition to taking preventive measures to avoid a crisis, a person with diabetes should have a social network in place for assistance in case of prolonged hypoglycemia.

Here are some suggestions:

- Ask a friend or relative to telephone every morning.
- Ask the mailman to deliver the mail in person.
- Agree on a code system with a neighbour (for example, one curtain open or closed upon waking).
- Use a personal response medical alert service with a two-way voice communication system such as Philips Lifeline: 514-735-2101 or 1 877 423-9700.

It is a good idea to leave a house key with a friend or relative who can help if necessary.

Can symptoms of hypoglycemia occur when blood glucose is normal?

Yes, there are two situations in which a person with diabetes can have symptoms of hypoglycemia when blood glucose is normal:

- When hyperglycemia has existed for some time, using antidiabetic medications to normalize blood glucose levels too quickly can trigger symptoms of hypoglycemia that can last up to several days. To avoid this unpleasant feeling, it may be necessary to slow down the treatment so that blood sugar can decrease more gradually. The ultimate goal is always to regain a normal blood glucose level.
- When blood glucose is quite elevated and then quickly drops back to normal, symptoms of hypoglycemia may appear and then

fade quickly. If you suspect hypoglycemia, always test your blood glucose levels, because treating a false case of hypoglycemia can cause hyperglycemia.

Is reactive hypoglycemia a sign of diabetes?

Sometimes. In some cases, reactive hypoglycemia is the first sign of type 2 diabetes. In such a case, the delayed drop in blood glucose levels is related to an excessive and delayed secretion of insulin caused by a carbohydrate-rich meal. This type of hypoglycemia usually appears three or four hours after such a meal – hence the term "reactive." In general, reactive hypoglycemia corrects itself spontaneously, even if no carbohydrates are ingested. The condition can be avoided by eating balanced meals, especially at breakfast and in snacks.

The symptoms or signs of hypoglycemia do not always occur simultaneously

---

The symptoms of hypoglycemia can differ from person to person.

Symptoms and discomforts can change over time. A person who has had diabetes for 10 to 20 years may no longer experience the symptoms of hypoglycemia (neuropathy).

The symptoms of hypoglycemia can be masked by certain medications such as beta-blockers.

The symptoms of hypoglycemia may be absent if the person suffers from repeated episodes.

Some of the symptoms of hypoglycemia are difficult to assess. Glucose levels should therefore be confirmed with a glucose meter to avoid unnecessary correction.

Hypoglycemia should be corrected immediately, following the recommended steps, to ensure that there is no damage to the brain or heart. There is no such thing as "minor hypoglycemia."

What precautions should be taken by a person with diabetes at risk of hypoglycemia when driving a vehicle?

Check your blood glucose before getting behind the wheel.

- If your blood glucose is higher than or equal to 5.0 mmol/L, it is safe to drive and no precautions are necessary.
- If your blood glucose is between 4.0 and 5.0 mmol/L before driving, have a snack with 15 g of carbohydrates and check your blood glucose fifteen minutes later.
- If your blood glucose is lower than 4.0 mmol/L, avoid driving and treat the hypoglycemia as recommended. Once your blood glucose has been higher than 5.0 mmol/L for at least 45 minutes, it is safe to take the wheel.
- Check your blood glucose every 4 hours of driving, and keep carbohydrate-based snacks on hand.

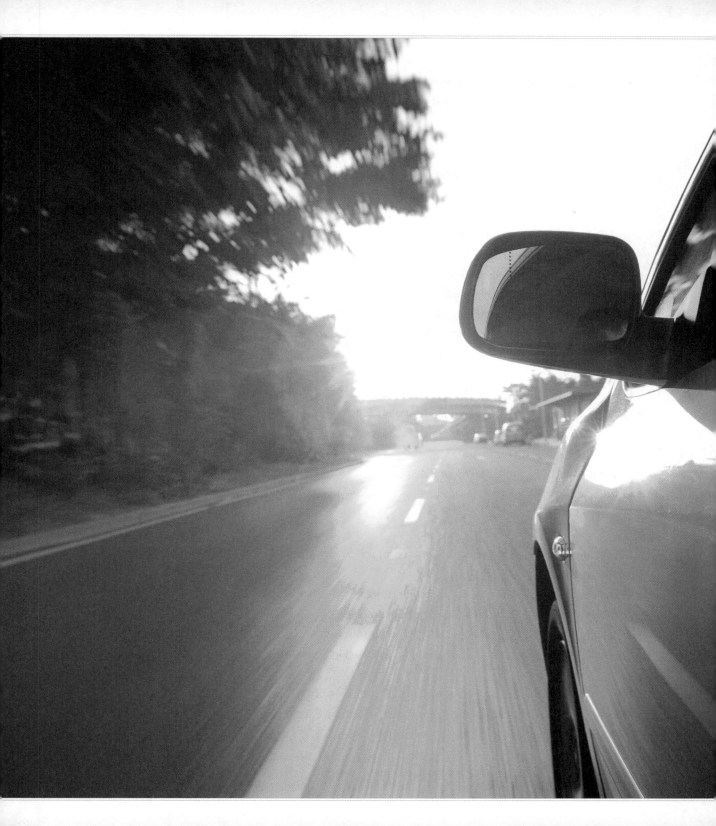

RECOMMENDATIONS FOR THE TREATMENT OF HYPOGLYCEMIA[1]
IN PEOPLE WITH DIABETES

Test blood glucose immediately

If blood glucose is lower than 4.0 mmol/L

MILD OR MODERATE HYPOGLYCEMIA

If no assistance is required for treatment, take 15 g of carbohydrates in one of the appropriate forms:

- 4 tablets of Dex4® (1 tablet = 4 g of carbohydrates)
- 59 mL of Dex4®C liquid (1 bottle = 16 g of carbohydrates)
- 5 tablets of Dextro® = (1 tablet = 3 g of carbohydrates)
- 7 tablets of Glucosol® (1 tablet = 2.25 g of carbohydrates)
- 15 mL (3 tsp, 3 packets, or 3 cubes) of sugar dissolved in water
- 15 mL (3 tsp) of maple or corn syrup

Other foods containing approximately 15 g of carbohydrates

- 125 to 175 mL (½ to ¾ cup) of regular (not diet) soda or fruit beverage
- 125 to 175 mL (½ to ¾ cup) of fruit juice, no sugar added
- 1 dry fruit bar (e.g., "Fruit to go")
- 1 small appel, ½ banana, 2 kiwis, or 2 dates, etc.
- 1 tube de Dex4® in gel form (1 tube = 17 g of carbohydrates)

SEVERE HYPOGLYCEMIA

If the person is conscious but needs assistance for treatment, give him or her 20 g of carbohydrates.
First choice (absorbed quickly)

- 5 tablets of Dex4® (1 tablet = 4 g of carbohydrates)
- 7 tablets of Dextro® (1 tablet = 3 g of carbohydrates)
- 9 tablets of Glucosol® (1 tablet = 2.25 g of carbohydrates)
- 20 mL (4 tsp, 4 packets, or 4 cubes) of sugar dissolved in water

Other choices containing approximately 20 g of carbohydrates

- 175 to 250 mL (¾ to 1 cup) of regular (not diet) soft drink or fruit beverage
- Tube of Insta-Glucose® (1 tube = 24 g of carbohydrates)

[1] Canadian Diabetes Association Clinical Practice Guidelines Expert Committee. Canadian Diabetes Association 2013 Clinical Practice Guidelines for the Prevention and Management of Diabetes in Canada. *Can. J. Diabetes* 2013;37(suppl 1):S1-S212

Wait 15 minutes to test blood glucose again

If blood glucose is still below 4.0 mmol/L, have another 15 g of carbohydrates

Wait 15 minutes and repeat treatment as needed

When blood glucose reaches or exceeds 4.0 mmol/L

Meal (or snack) expected within one hour or less

YES	NO
Have the meal or snack as planned	Have a snack containing 15 g of carbohydrates and a protein source (e.g., 200 mL of milk and 2 dry Social Tea biscuits) while waiting for the meal

If the person is unconscious

- Inject 1 mg glucagon subcutaneously (under the skin) or intramuscularly (dose for adults and children weighing more than 20 kg or 44 lb).
- When the person regains consciousness and is able to swallow, provide a meal or a normal snack according to the regular schedule to prevent hyperglycemia. If the next meal is more than an hour away, provide a snack of 45 g of carbohydrates with a protein source.

CAUTION

1. People with diabetes taking acarbose (Glucobay®) in combination with other medications that may cause hypoglycemia should correct their hypoglycemia in one of the following ways:
- 4 tablets of Dex4® (1 tablet = 4 g of carbohydrates) or
- 5 tablets of Dextro® (1 tablet = 3 g of carbohydrates) or
- 300 mL (1 ¼ cup) of milk

2. People with diabetes suffering from kidney damage should correct their hypoglycemia in one of the following ways:
- 4 tablets of Dex4® (1 tablet = 4 g of carbohydrates) or
- 5 tablets of Dextro® (1 tablet = 3 g of carbohydrates) or
- 15 mL (3 tsp, 3 packets, or 3 cubes) of sugar dissolved in a bit of water

3. Hypoglycemia should never be dismissed as minor or unimportant. All appropriate measures should be taken to prevent it. When it occurs, it should be treated immediately.

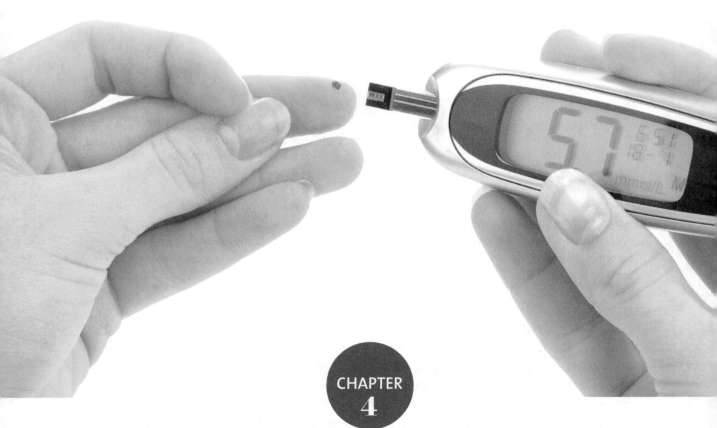

Self-monitoring:
Blood Glucose and
Glycated Hemoglobin (A1C)

What is self-monitoring?

Self-monitoring is a technique used by people with diabetes to **measure their own blood glucose levels**. By extension, the approach usually includes adjusting treatment based on the results obtained to bring and maintain blood glucose levels as close to normal as possible.

Why is it important to self-monitor?

Self-monitoring lets people with diabetes:

- measure the impact of **nutrition**, **physical activity**, **stress** and **antidiabetic drugs** on their blood glucose;
- identify episodes of hypoglycemia and hyperglycemia and react quickly;
- modify their behaviour with respect to nutrition, physical activity, antidiabetic drugs and stress, if necessary;
- measure the impact of these changes on their blood glucose;
- feel confident, safe, and independent in the management of their diabetes; and above all,
- bring and maintain blood glucose levels as close to normal as possible.

Why should people with diabetes try to maintain blood glucose levels as close to normal as possible?

People with diabetes should try to maintain their blood glucose levels as close as possible to normal to prevent complications associated with diabetes.

Two major studies (one American study on type 1 diabetes and one British study on type 2 diabetes) have shown that maintaining blood glucose levels as close to normal as possible significantly **reduces the development and progression of microvascular complications due to diabetes**. The results showed:

- a decrease in **retinopathy** of 21% to 76%
- a decrease in **nephropathy** of 34% to 54%
- a decrease in **neuropathy** of 40% to 60% or an improvement in the existing neuropathy.

How is blood glucose measured from the fingertip?

A glucose meter is used to measure blood glucose in blood taken from the fingertip. The procedure involves two steps:

PREPARE THE MATERIALS AND CHECK THE REAGENT STRIPS

- **Wash your hands** with soapy water and dry them thoroughly. This reduces the risk of infection and makes it easier to take the blood sample. Alcohol swabs are not recommended for home use because they can dry out the skin, which can lead to cracked fingertips.

- **Prepare the material:** meter, test strip, holder, lancet, paper tissue.
- **Insert the lancet into the lancing device** and set it. Never use a lancet more than once, and do not throw it directly in the trash. You can pick up special medical waste containers at no charge at a pharmacy or community health centre. Once the container is full, return it for safe disposal. Never use a lancet or a holder that another person has already used.
- Check the reagent strip container for the manufacturer's expiration date.
- When you open a container for the first time, write the date on it to **keep track of the life expectancy of the strips.**
- **Take out a test strip.** If the strip comes from a vial, close the vial immediately.

ANALYZE THE BLOOD AND RECORD THE DATA

- Power on the device, if necessary.
- Insert the test strip into the strip support on the meter or automatically release a strip from the device.
- Prick the lateral extremity (side of the tip) of a finger. Switch sides and fingers every time you take a blood sample.
- Produce a **large drop of blood** by applying pressure on the finger while pointing it downwards. Do not press too hard.
- Place the **first drop of blood** on the reactive part of the strip or, depending on the type of meter, bring the reactive part of the strip into contact with the blood.

- Wait for the reading to be displayed.
- **Enter the result** in the appropriate column of your self-monitoring logbook.

Can blood from any other part of the body be used to measure blood glucose?

Blood glucose can be measured with blood drawn from alternate sites such as the forearm, the arm, the palm, the abdomen or the thigh.

Several glucose meters now offer this option.

Results from alternative sites are generally comparable to glucose readings taken from the fingertip before a meal. This method of measuring blood glucose has some limits, however, and it is recommended that a blood glucose reading be taken from the fingertip in situations where blood glucose can fluctuate rapidly, such as:

- during an episode of hypoglycemia;
- during physical activity;
- up to two hours after a meal;
- immediately after an insulin injection;
- during an illness.

Which glucose meters are currently available, and what are their features?

The tables on pages 48 to 53 list the latest generation of glucose meters on the market, along with some of their features (list updated on May 1, 2013).

Glucose meters are frequently offered for free, and many manufacturers will trade new meters for old ones at no cost. Continuous glucose monitors can cost as much as $2,000.

Strips cost between $0.50 and $1.00 each. There are special offers on some strips, and prices can vary from one pharmacy to another.

What are the main causes of false glucose readings?

False readings occur primarily when:
- the glucose meter is dirty;
- the glucose meter is calibrated incorrectly;
- the user forgets to calibrate the meter, leaving out the calibration code for the current batch of reagent strips;
- the strips have expired;
- the strips have been exposed to humidity;
- the strips have been exposed to extreme temperatures;
- the drop of blood is too small;
- the user's technique is faulty (e.g., the time of contact with the strip is too short);
- the glucose meter is inaccurate.

How are glucose meters measured for accuracy?

The accuracy of readings from a glucose meter should be checked annually. The **fasting blood glucose** level from a laboratory blood test should be compared with the level obtained from the glucose meter. Blood glucose should be tested with the meter **within five minutes** after the blood sample is taken for the laboratory test.

The new 2013 ISO standards for blood glucose monitors stipulate that:
- for levels lower than 5.55 mmol/L, 95% of blood glucose readings must fall within 0.83 mmol/L of the reference reading;
- for levels equal to or higher than 5.55 mmol/L, 95% of blood glucose readings must be within 15% of the reference results.

HOW ARE GLUCOSE METERS MEASURED FOR ACCURACY?

Fasting

- Go for a blood test to have your "fasting blood glucose" measured in a lab.
- Within five minutes, take a fasting glucose reading with your meter as usual.
- Enter this result in the logbook and circle it.
- Ask for the results of the blood test the next time you visit your doctor.
- Calculate the accuracy of the meter.

	Example	Your results
Fasting blood glucose (lab test from blood sample)	10 mmol/L	
Blood glucose reading from fingertip with meter (taken within 5 minutes)	9.2 mmol/L	
Accuracy of meter expressed as a percentage	8%	

FORMULA TO CALCULATE ACCURACY OF METER

Example:

9.2
Blood glucose from fingertip with meter

Your result

(−)

10.0
Fasting blood glucose from blood test

Your result

(÷)

10.0
Fasting blood glucose from blood test

Your result

(x) **100** (=) %

A variation of 15% or less is considered acceptable.

Aim for a smaller variation for blood glucose levels below 5.55 mmol/L.

New 2013 ISO standard.

How often should blood glucose levels be measured?[1]

Self-monitoring should be adapted to the individual's situation.

1 TYPE 1 OR TYPE 2

Generally, people using the **insulin pump** and people with type 1 or type 2 diabetes taking **4 or more daily injections** should measure their blood glucose at least *4 times a day*.

Your doctor may also ask you to take a reading two hours after meals (generally, begin counting the time after your first mouthful) and even during the night.

2 TYPE 2

Generally, the recommendations for people with type 2 diabetes are the following:

- If you take **less than 4 daily injections** of insulin, take *at least one blood glucose reading for every injection*.
- If you take **secretagogues** (drugs known to cause hypoglycemia by stimulating insulin secretion), take a reading when the *symptoms of hypoglycemia* occur or *at specific times* that those symptoms have occurred whether or not symptoms are currently present.

- If you take antidiabetic medications that **do not cause a risk of hypoglycemi**a or if you treat your diabetes with lifestyle modification (nutrition, physical activity, stress management), take a reading *once or twice a week* to be sure you are reaching your blood glucose targets.

3 PREGNANCY

In general, it is recommended that women with diabetes who **want to become pregnant** or who **are pregnant** (whether or not they are on insulin therapy) tailor their self-monitoring to their specific situation. They may need to measure blood glucose *4 times or more* every day.

4 NEW DIAGNOSIS

In general, it is recommended that people who have been **diagnosed with diabetes within the last six months** measure their blood glucose *once a day at different times* (before each meal and before the evening snack) to understand the effects that meals, physical activity, stress, and medication can have on their blood glucose.

Generally, people who **attain their blood glucose targets** through lifestyle modifications are **not required to take daily readings**.

---

1 Adapted from Canadian Diabetes Association Clinical Practice Guidelines Expert Committee, Canadian Diabetes Association. 2013 Clinical Practice Guidelines for the Prevention and Management of Diabetes in Canada. *Can. J. Diabetes* 2013; 37(suppl 1): S1-S212.

5 PREDIABETES

Generally, people with prediabetes **do not need to take daily readings**.

6 SPECIFIC SITUATIONS

There are **specific situations** where people with diabetes are generally advised to measure their blood glucose more frequently at various times of the day:

- When **adjusting treatment**, take at least two readings a day until targets are reached.
- When **any discomfort** suggesting hypoglycemia or hyperglycemia is experienced, take a reading.
- When making **any change** in nutrition, physical activity, stress, or medication, increase the frequency.
- When **driving a vehicle,** take a reading before taking the wheel and every four hours during long trips to prevent hypoglycemia.
- When **exercising**, take a reading before, during and after the activity to prevent hypoglycemia;
- When **taking new medications** that can cause hyperglycemia (e.g., cortisone), self-monitoring should be tailored to your situation. You might need to take two or more readings daily.
- If you are doing **work** that absolutely requires that you avoid an episode of hypoglycemia, take a blood glucose reading as often as necessary.
- When suffering from an **illness** known to cause hyperglycemia (e.g., an infection), self-monitoring should be tailored to your situation. You might need to take two or more readings daily.
- When **hospitalized** or when suffering from an acute illness, self-monitoring should be tailored to your situation. You might need to take four or more readings daily.

What information should be recorded in the logbook to make blood glucose control as easy as possible?

Blood glucose control is easier when the following information is recorded in the logbook:

- the result and date of **blood glucose** readings (in the column corresponding to the meal: e.g. "Before lunch");
- relevant comments such as the reason for the **hypoglycemia**, any change in diet, any physical activity, etc.;
- the result of a **ketone bodies** reading from urine or blood, with the date and time (in the "Comments" column);
- the name, dose and time of ingestion of **all prescribed antidiabetic drugs**; write down every change or omission in the "Comments" column;
- the quantity of carbohydrates consumed in meals and snacks;
- the area of the insulin injection, if applicable, the technique used, and so on (in the "Comments" column).

11

How should the information be recorded?

The information should be noted in the **self-monitoring logbook**. Group information of the same nature together in a clearly identified column:

- In the first column, enter the results of blood glucose readings taken **before breakfast** over the course of a single week.
- In the second column, enter the results of blood glucose readings taken **after breakfast** over the course of a single week.
- In the next columns, do the same with the results of the **other blood glucose readings** taken before and after lunch and dinner, before bedtime (before a snack), and during the night.
- **Hypoglycemia** occurring outside the four usual glucose reading periods should be noted in the following period (e.g., hypoglycemia occurring in the afternoon should be entered in the column corresponding to "Before dinner").
- Unmeasured hypoglycemia should be assigned a reading of **2mmol/L**.
- **Weekly average** glucose readings should be entered at the bottom of each column (do not include the results of hypoglycemic correction when calculating the average). See the example marked by two asterisks (**) in the table on the next page.
- When calculating averages, do not include readings associated with an exceptional, isolated, and explainable situation; see the example marked by an asterisk (*) in the table on the next page.
- Enter any relevant remarks in the "Comments" column.

EXAMPLE OF A SELF-MONITORING LOGBOOK

Week beginning on Sunday: 01 (day) 05 (month) 2013 (year)

Day of the week	Blood glucose results (mmol/L)							Comments
	Breakfast		Lunch		Dinner		Bedtime	
	Before	After	Before	After	Before	After	Before snack	
Sunday	5.2		12.1					
Monday	7.1				8.1			
Tuesday	4.6						4.1	
Wednesday	9.3		10.4			12.3		
Thursday	5.5				7.2		6.7	
Friday	6.8				3.5*		16.6**	* Exercise ** Corrected hypoglycemia
Saturday	3.9		11.3		18.1*			*Stress
Average	6.1		11.3		7.7		5.4	

The average is calculated by adding all the numbers from the same column and dividing the total by the number of entries in the column. For example, the average blood glucose before lunch is calculated as follows:

$$(12.1 + 10.4 + 11.3) \div 3 = 33.8 \div 3 = 11.3$$

Will the doctor prescribe any other tests in addition to blood glucose readings to monitor blood glucose control?

In addition to blood glucose readings, the doctor may prescribe blood tests to measure **glycated hemoglobin** (A1C) and in some cases fructosamine. These two laboratory tests indicate how well the diabetes has been managed.

GLYCATED HEMOGLOBIN, OR A1C

The level of glycated hemoglobin (A1C) reflects how well blood glucose has been controlled over the last two to three months.

This type of hemoglobin forms when glucose (sugar) in the blood binds with the hemoglobin in red blood cells. The higher the blood glucose, the more sugar molecules bind with hemoglobin and raise A1C levels.

A blood test is used to measure A1C. It should be done two to four times a year, depending on how well the diabetes is managed. The A1C value is essential information, as it can provide an overall picture blood glucose control and enable treatment adjustments.

The A1C test is complementary to blood glucose readings. It does not indicate blood glucose variations, hypoglycemia, or hyperglycemia. The generally recommended target is an A1C value of 7% (0.070) or less. For some patients with type 2 diabetes, a target A1C equal to or less than 6.5% (0.065) may be targeted to reduce the risk of kidney damage even more. This type of stricter control should be done carefully, taking into account any possibility of hypoglycaemia and any risk to cardiovascular health.

For some people with diabetes who are more vulnerable (due to age, long-standing diabetes, complications, or other diseases), the target glycated hemoglobin may be as high as 8.5%.

FRUCTOSAMINE

Fructosamine levels reflect how well blood glucose has been controlled over the last two to three weeks.

The practice of using fructosamine levels as a marker of the risk of complications of diabetes is not as well established. Nevertheless, this type of reading, which is performed with a blood test, can be useful in some cases. For example, it can be used:

- for a short-term assessment of a change in treatment;
- for an assessment of blood glucose management when A1C levels are less reliable (e.g., in the case of hemoglobin disease or severe anemia);
- for a follow-up on blood glucose control during pregnancy.

A normal fructosamine level is generally between 200 and 290 µmol/L. Like A1C, fructosamine does not indicate blood glucose variations and is used as a complement to regular blood glucose readings.

NON-EXHAUSTIVE LIST OF GLUCOSE METERS (UPDATED ON MAY 1, 2013)

GLUCOSE METER	MANUFACTURER	RANGE OF RESULTS (MMOL/L)	TEMPERATURE RANGE OF STRIPS (°C)	
FreeStyle InsuLinx	Abbott	1.1 to 27.8	4°C to 40°C	
FreeStyle Lite	Abbott	1.1 to 27.8	4°C to 40°C	
Precision Xtra Blood glucose (G) Ketone bodies (K)	Abbott	G : 1.1 to 27.8 K: 0 to 8.0	15°C to 40°C	
Contour Next EZ	Bayer	0.6 to 33.3	0°C to 30°C	
Contour Next USB	Bayer	1.1 to 33.3	0°C to 30°C	
OneTouch Verio IQ	LifeScan	1.1 to 33.3	6°C to 44°C	
OneTouch Ultra 2	LifeScan	1.1 to 33.3	6°C to 44°C	
OneTouch UltraMini	LifeScan	1.1 to 33.3	6°C to 44°C	
Medi+Sure	Medi+Sure Canada	1.1 to 41.7	10°C to 40°C	
Guardian REAL-Time	Medtronic MiniMed	2.2 to 22.2	N/A	
Nova Max Plus Blood glucose (G) Ketone bodies (K)	Nova Biomedical	G: 1.1 to 33.3 K: 0.1 to 8.0	15°C to 39°C	
Accu-Check Aviva Nano	Roche Diagnostics	0.6 to 33.3	10°C to 40°C	
Accu-Check Compact Plus	Roche Diagnostics	0.6 to 33.3	10°C to 40°C	
Accu-Check Mobile	Roche Diagnostics	0.6 to 33.3	10°C to 32°C	
BGStar and iBGStar	Sanofi	1.1 to 33.3	8°C to 30°C	
Oracle	Tremblay Harrison	1.1 to 33.3	10°C to 40°C	

CALIBRATION OF REAGENT STRIPS	LIFESPAN OF REAGENT STRIPS	REAGENT STRIPS
Automatic	Date on vial	Vial (sensitive to humidity)
Automatic	Date on vial	Vial (sensitive to humidity)
Calibrating strip in each box	Date on package	Individually wrapped
Automatic	Date on vial	Vial (sensitive to humidity)
Automatic	Date on vial	Vial (sensitive to humidity)
Automatic	6 months (after opening)	Vial (sensitive to humidity)
Calibrate to code 25	6 months (after opening)	Vial (sensitive to humidity)
Automatic	6 months (after opening)	N/A
Automatic	3 months (after opening)	Vial
N/A	Lifespan of sensor: 3 days	N/A
Automatic	3 months (after opening)	Vial
Code chip in each box	Date on vial	Vial (sensitive to humidity)
Automatic	3 months (after opening)	Cartridge of 17 strips
Automatic	3 months (after opening)	Box of 50 tests
Automatic	Date on vial	Vial (sensitive to humidity)
Automatic	3 months (after opening)	Vial (sensitive to humidity)

GLUCOSE METER	SOFTWARE AND NUMBER OF TESTS IN MEMORY	LANCING DEVICE	LANCETS	TELEPHONE ASSISTANCE	
FreeStyle InsuLinx	FreeStyle Auto-Assist 990	FreeStyle	FreeStyle 25 gauge	1-800-359-2606	
FreeStyle Lite	CoPilot 400	FreeStyle	FreeStyle 25 gauge	1-800-359-2606	
Precision Xtra Blood glucose (G) Ketone bodies (C)	CoPilot 450	Easy Touch Precision	Precision 28 gauge	1-800 359-2606	
Contour Next Ez	GLUCOFACTS DELUXE 480	Microlet 2	Microlet 28 gauge	1-800-268-7200	
Contour Next USB	GLUCOFACTS DELUXE 2000	Microlet 2	Microlet 28 gauge	1-800-268-7200	
OneTouch Verio IQ	OneTouch DMS 750 results 50 trends	One Touch Delica	One Touch Delica 33 gauge	1-800-663-5521	
OneTouch Ultra2	OneTouch 500	One Touch Delica	One Touch Delica 33 gauge	1-800-663-5521	
OneTouch UltraMini	OneTouch 500	One Touch Delica	One Touch Delica 33 gauge	1-800-663-5521	
Medi+Sure	Medi+Sure 960	SteriLance	SteriLance 28 and 33 gauge	1-855-634-7873	
Guardian REAL-Time	CareLink 288 readings/day 21 days of information	N/A	N/A	1-866-444-4649	

WEBSITE	SPECIFIC FEATURES
www.abbottdiabetescare.ca	• Tactile screen with backlight • Short-acting insulin calculator • Possibility of marking events before and after meals • Sending of daily data from the reader (option)
www.abbottdiabetescare.ca	• Possibility of adding blood for up to 60 seconds • Illuminated controls
www.abbottdiabetescare.ca	• Individually wrapped strips • Does not start if strips expired • Hematocrit range from 20% to 65-70% • Ketone body alert
www.bayerdiabetes.ca	• Simple features • Marking results before and after meals • Large, easy-to-read screen
www.bayerdiabetes.ca	• Carbohydrate and insulin values can be recorded • Marking of results before and after meals • USB connector
www.onetouch.ca	• Marking events before and after meals • Management of high or low blood glucose tendencies
www.onetouch.ca	• Marking of events before and after meals • DoubleSure technology (measures each sample twice instead of once) • Backlit screen
www.onetouch.ca	• DoubleSure technology (measures each sample twice instead of once) • Simple features
www.medisure.ca	• Strips 35 % cheaper
www.guardianrealtime.ca	• Continuous monitor for $2000 plus 5 sensors for $325 (3-day lifespan of sensor) • Alarm for hypo- or hyperglycemia • Not water-resistant

GLUCOSE METER	SOFTWARE AND NUMBER OF TESTS IN MEMORY	LANCING DEVICE	LANCETS	
Nova Max Plus Blood glucose (G) Ketone bodies (K)	CD Nova Max Connect 400	Nova	Nova automatic 33 gauge	
Accu-Check Aviva Nano	Accu-Check 360 or Smart Pix 500	Accu-Check Softclix	Accu-Check Softclix lancets 28 gauge	
Accu-Check Compact Plus	Accu-Check 360 or Smart Pix 500	Accu-Check Softclix	Individual Accu-Check Softclix lancets 28 gauge	
Accu-Check Mobile	Accu-Check 360 or Smart Pix 500	Accu-Check Fastclix Mobile	Cartridge of 6 Accu-Check Fastclix lancets 30 gauge	
BGStar and iBGStar	• iBGStar: iPhone or iPod Touch app • BGStar: 1865 • iBGStar: 300 but unlimited when connected to iPhone or iPod Touch	BGStar	BGStar 33 gauge	
Oracle	EZ Health Oracle 450 management software	Oracle	Oracle 30 gauge	

Glucose meters take between 4 and 6 seconds for analysis and the amount of blood needed varies between 0.3 and 1.5 mL. Ask the manufacturer if your glucose meter comples with the new 2013 ISO standard.

TELEPHONE ASSISTANCE	WEBSITE	SPECIFIC FEATURES
1-800-260-1021	www.novacares.ca	• Glucose and ketone body level readings
1-800-363-7949	www.accu-check.ca	• Wide strips • Hypoglycemia indicator • Post-meal test reminder • Circle of Care program
1-800-363-7949	www.accu-check.ca	• Backlit screen • All-in-one: meter, strips and lancing device • Audio beep for vision-impaired • Circle of Care program
1-800-363-7949	www.accu-check.ca	• Backlit screen • All-in-one: meter, strips and lancing device • Circle of Care program
1-888-852-6887	www.starsystem.sanofi.ca	• Average before and after meals • Typical variations • Graphics on iBGStar screen • Hypo- and hyperglycia alarm and reminder alarm • STARsystem program and health coaching
1-866-829-7926	www.oraclediabetes.com	• Voice function for vision impaired (English and French)

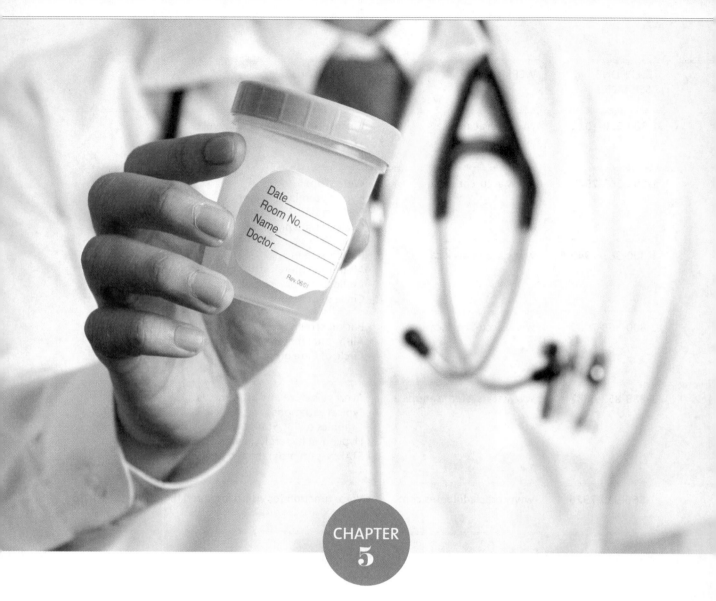

CHAPTER
5

Measuring
Ketone Bodies[1]

What are ketone bodies?

Ketone bodies are **by-products of the breakdown of body fat.**

What does an increase of ketone bodies in the blood mean?

An increase of ketone bodies in the blood indicates that a **lack of insulin** is causing a person with diabetes to use **fat** reserves stored in the body instead of **glucose.**

Without insulin, many cells in the body are unable to use glucose in the blood. When the body lacks insulin, it uses energy stored in the form of fat, and the breakdown of this fat leads to the production of **ketone bodies.** Ketone bodies are acids, and their presence can lead to **diabetic ketoacidosis.**

Excess ketone bodies in the blood are eliminated through the urine. As a result, they can be measured in either blood or urine.

Why should people with diabetes check for excess ketone bodies in blood or urine?

People with diabetes—especially type 1—should check for excess ketone bodies in blood or urine **because an excess indicates poor management of the disease** and a risk of diabetic

ketoacidosis, which can lead to coma. In some cases, doctors recommend this type of monitoring for people with type 2 diabetes.

When should people with diabetes check for ketone bodies in blood or urine?

Blood or urine should be tested for ketone bodies when **blood glucose** is **higher than 14 mmol/L or when a doctor recommends it.**

The test should be repeated, along with four (or more, if necessary) blood glucose readings a day, until there are no excess **ketone bodies** in the blood or urine and **blood glucose** is **back whitin target range.**

Blood or urine should also be tested for ketone bodies if the following symptoms are experienced:
- intense thirst;
- abdominal pain;
- excessive tiredness or drowsiness;
- nausea and vomiting.

---

1 Canadian Diabetes Association Clinical Practice Guidelines Expert Committee. Canadian Diabetes Association 2013 Clinical Practice Guidelines for the Prevention and Management of Diabetes in Canada. *Can. J. Diabetes 2013*; 37(suppl 1):S1-S212.

What should be done if excess ketone bodies are detected in the blood or urine?

A person with diabetes who finds excess ketone bodies in the blood or urine should:

1 **drink 250 mL of water** every hour to hydrate and help eliminate ketone bodies through the urine;

2 **take extra doses of insulin (Humalog®, NovoRapid®, Apidra®, Humulin®R or Novolin® ge Toronto)** according to doctor's recommendations (*see chapter 21, page 196 on Hyperglycemic Emergencies*);

3 call a doctor **immediately** or go to the emergency room if there is a persistent excess of ketone bodies in the blood or urine despite treatment, and if the following symptoms appear:

- abdominal pain;
- excessive tiredness or drowsiness;
- nausea and vomiting.

How are ketone bodies measured in urine?

Ketone bodies in urine can be measured with Ketostix®, a reagent strip. There are also reagent strips that measure glucose and ketone bodies in the urine simultaneously (e.g., Chemstrip® uG/K, Keto-Diastix®).

PREPARE THE MATERIAL

With Ketostix®:

1 Gather the material: Ketostix® reagent strips, a clean and dry container, and a timer.

2 Check the manufacturer's expiry date on the reagent strip container. When opening the container for the first time, write the date on the container. It must be discarded six months after being opened.

Ketostix® reagent strips should be stored at room temperature (between 15°C and 30°C).

3 Collect a **fresh** urine sample for analysis:

- Empty the bladder completely and discard the urine.
- Drink one or two glasses of water.
- Urinate into a clean, dry container.

4 Take a reagent strip from the container and close the cover **immediately**.

Compare the colour of the reagent strip with the chart on the container to be certain that the strip has not changed colour, as this could give a false result.

Test the urine sample with the reagent strip

1 Dip the reactive part of the strip into the fresh urine sample and remove it right away.

2 Tap the excess fluid off the strip on the edge of the container and start the timer

Note: Instructions for reading the results and storing the strips can vary from brand to brand. Read them carefully.

Read and record the result

1 After **exactly 15 seconds**, place the reagent strip next to the colour chart on the strip container and compare the result under a bright light.
2 Enter the result in your glucose self-monitoring logbook.

Negative	Trace	Low	Moderate	High
0	0.5 mmol/L	1.5 mmol/L	4 mmol/L	From 8 mmol/L to 16 mmol/L

How are ketone bodies measured in a fingertip blood sample?

Ketone bodies in the blood are measured with a ketone meter, either the Nova Max® Plus™ or the Precision Xtra®.

PREPARE THE MATERIAL

1 Gather the material: meter (to measure blood glucose and ketone bodies), reagent strips for measuring ketonemia (detectable ketone bodies), lancing device, lancet.
2 Check the expiry date on the reagent strip envelope.
3 **Precision Xtra®**: Insert the ketone calibrator in the meter. The code displayed on the screen must match the code on the reagent strip.
   Nova Max® Plus™: No calibration is necessary.

4 Insert the ketone strip into the Precision Xtra® meter.

APPLY THE BLOOD SAMPLE TO THE REAGENT STRIP

Precision Xtra®:

1 Prick the fingertip with the lancing device.
2 Apply a drop of blood to the reactive area of the strip.

Read and record the result

1 Wait for the result to appear on the screen; it should appear within 10 seconds.
2 Enter the result in the self-monitoring log-book.

Note: If using the Nova Max® Plus™, refer to the manufacturer's instructions included with the product.

Negative	Trace	Low	Moderate	High
0	Less than 0.6 mmol/L	From 0.6 mmol/L to 1.5 mmol/L	From 1.5 mmol/L to 3 mmol/L	Over 3 mmol/L

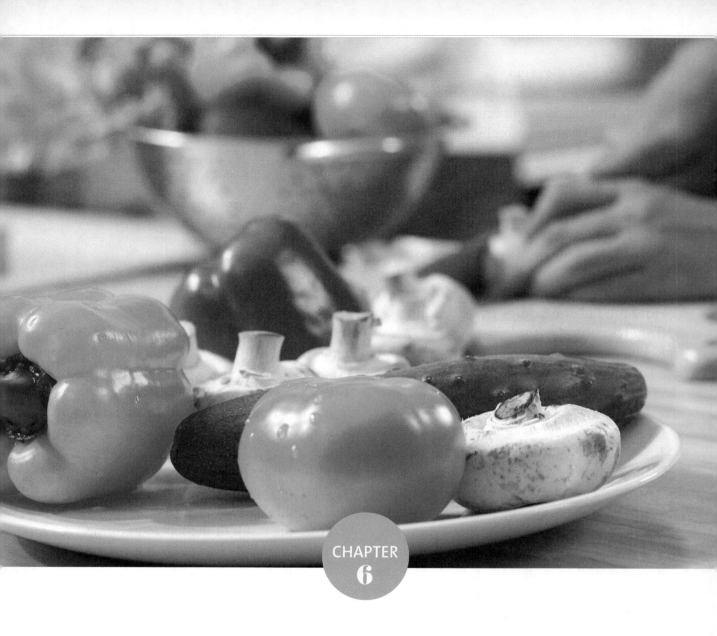

Eating Well

Why is it important for people with diabetes to eat well?

Eating well is part of a wholesome routine that promotes good health and the better management of diabetes. What and how much you eat are important decisions, and making informed choices can help you meet your body's real needs.

The main characteristics of a healthy diet is variety and balance, not restrictions or prohibitions.

Whether or not you take oral antidiabetic medications or insulin, your diet will always be an integral and important part of your treatment.

What are the benefits of a healthy diet?

A healthy diet:

1 promotes better control of:
- blood glucose;
- weight;
- blood pressure;
- blood lipids (fats).
2 fulfills the body's energy (calories), vitamin and mineral requirements;
3 promotes well-being.

What foods should be preferred?

People with diabetes, just like everyone else, should follow the recommendations in *Eating Well with Canada's Food Guide*.

- Eat at least one dark green and one orange vegetable every day; choose fresh fruit or vegetables instead of juice.
- Eat at least half of the recommended grain products in the form of whole grains.
- Drink skim, 1% or 2% milk or enriched soya beverages every day.
- Eat meat alternatives such as legumes and tofu often.
- Eat at least two portions of fish per week.
- Eat a small amount of good, unsaturated fats (such as olive oil or canola oil) every day.
- Drink water to quench your thirst.

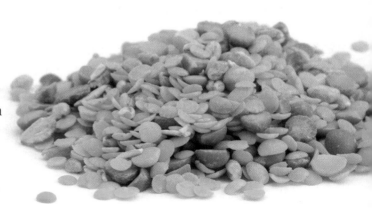

How can diet help control blood glucose?

People with diabetes maintain better control of their blood glucose if:

- they take their meals at the same time every day. This is particularly true for people with diabetes taking oral antidiabetic drugs that stimulate insulin secretion (for example, Diaßeta®) and those taking insulin. It can also decrease the occurrence of large variations in blood glucose levels such as hyperglycemia or hypoglycemia.
- they spread out their calories and in particular their carbohydrates evenly over at least three meals spaced four to six hours apart, and never skip a meal.
- they eat a moderate amount of carbohydrates in meals (and, if necessary, between meals) that corresponds to their energy needs. Carbohydrates are essential, but too many can hamper proper blood glucose management and cause hyperglycemia.
- the carbohydrate content of each meal is consistent from one day to the next.

Other aspects and components of nutrients – the glycemic index, dietary fibre, added sugar, proteins, and fats – can also affect blood glucose levels. These will be discussed in the following chapters.

How does losing weight affect blood glucose control?

The improvement of blood glucose control through weight loss is a treatment objective for overweight people (BMI over 24.9[1]). Moderate weight loss – between 5% and 10% of your starting weight – can improve insulin sensitivity, blood glucose control, blood pressure, and blood lipids.

Are there any diets that can help control blood glucose?

In addition to the traditional approach based on *Canada's Food Guide*, other diets have been recognized to have a positive impact on weight, blood lipids, blood pressure, and blood glucose control. The choice of approach is first and foremost a matter of personal values and preferences.

The Mediterranean diet is high in plant-based foods, including fruit, vegetables, legumes, nuts, grains, unrefined cereals, and moderate amounts of olive oil as a main source of fat, as well as small to moderate amounts of dairy products, fish and poultry, small amounts of red meat, and small to moderate amounts of red wine with meals. This way of eating has been shown to be an effective way of improving blood glucose control, lowering the risk of cardiovascular disease, and reducing blood pressure and the occurrence of cardiovascular events.

The **DASH diet** (Dietary Approaches to Stop Hypertension) is an approach that favours fruit, vegetables, and low-fat dairy products, but also includes whole grains, poultry, fish and nuts, as well as small amounts of red meat, cold cuts, and sweetened foods. This diet has been shown to be an effective way of losing weight, improving blood glucose control, and lowering blood pressure.

The vegetarian diet, frequently lower in fats and calories, has been shown to be an effective way of lowering A1C, weight, and cholesterol. A nutritionist can help choose foods to ensure that the diet is sufficient and rule out any deficiencies (e.g., vitamin B12).

Whatever the diet, people who are overweight should limit their calorie consumption slightly so that they can lose weight gradually and keep it off. Portion control is a necessary aspect of a weight-loss diet.

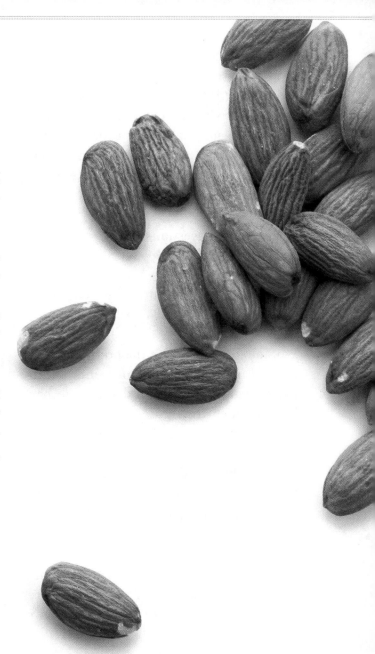

1 This measurement applies to people under the age of 65. People who are 65 and over are considered obese when their BMI is higher than 30.

How do I control how much I eat?

Eating well also involves choosing **the amounts of food you need**. That means eating to satisfy your hunger, but no more.[2] This is an interesting concept that can help you make lasting changes to the way you eat.

Here are a few suggestions:[3]

- **Get back in touch with your physical sensations** to learn how to tell the difference between physiological and psychological hunger.

Physiological hunger is the body's need for nourishment (fuel and nutrients), while psychological hunger is a defence mechanism in which the desire to eat is a way of dealing with uncontrollable emotions.

Learning how to distinguish between these two types of hunger is the first, indispensable step to being able to eat without excess or frustration.

The next step is to learn how to recognize the feeling of fullness. This task requires constant effort, patience, and perseverance.

Here is a little trick: try not to eat anything at all for four hours. This can help you remember what hunger feels like, learn how to identify it, and gradually re-establish a healthy relationship with food.

- **Establish a routine:** Have a similar breakfast every morning and eat your meals at the same times every day. This will help you feel physically hungry just before mealtime and full after eating.
- **Focus on taste:** Pay particular attention, taking small bites, chewing well, and savouring the food.
- **Slow down:** Take at least 20 minutes to eat a meal. This will give your stomach the time it needs to send fullness signals to the brain. Putting your knife and fork down between each bite can help you pace yourself.
- **Take a break in the middle of the meal:** This will give you a chance to assess whether you are still hungry. If eating has become less enjoyable, you have had enough.
- **Avoid distractions.** Just eat. Don't read the newspaper, watch television, or have an animated conversation. It may be helpful to take frequent breaks during the meal to talk and listen; this can ensure that you remain focussed and do only one thing at a time
- **Identify cravings:** Ask yourself whether your appetite is being triggered by something besides a physiological need or real hunger. If it is just a craving, take the time to figure out what emotions you are feeling and write them down in a journal.
- **Don't overeat now for later:** The desire to stockpile "just in case" and the fear of "not having enough" later are frequent consequences of restrictive diets. Come back to the present, and ask yourself how hungry you are right now.

- **Be your own judge:** Tune in to your own needs instead of eating to please someone else or to avoid giving offence. You alone should decide how much food you should eat.

Does eating well mean never eating cold cuts, French fries, chips or pastries?

These foods can be a part of a healthy diet. While it is true that they are often high in fat, sugar and calories, excluding them from your diet altogether can be a mistake, especially if you want to lose weight. Depriving yourself of a certain type of food merely increases your desire for it and leads to overindulgence. It is better to give yourself permission to enjoy a few chips once in a while instead of developing an uncontrollable craving and eating a whole bag. In this way, these foods can play a small role in a balanced diet and can be eaten on occasion, simply for the pleasure they give.[4]

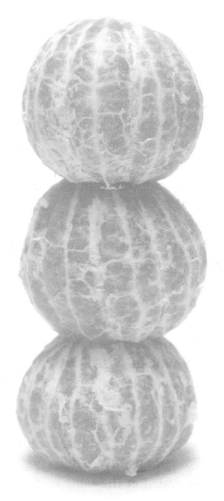

Are snacks necessary?

Many people make snacks between meals a requirement as a way of better controlling their blood sugar. While they are not strictly necessary, snacks can be included in a meal plan to help a person eat fewer carbohydrates at meals, spreading them out evenly over the course of the day, with a view to managing blood glucose more efficiently.

2 Apfeldorfer G. *Maigrir, c'est fou* (Odile Jacob, 2000), 301 pages.
3 Collectif 2007, *"Retrouver le plaisir de manger"* Psychologies, special edition, No. 9.
4 Groupe Équilibre : www.equilibre.ca

How can eating well help manage blood pressure?

Choose a diet rich in:

- fruit and vegetables, either fresh or frozen (rich in potassium and magnesium);
- low-fat dairy products (rich in calcium);
- soluble dietary fibre, as in legumes, oatmeal and oat bran;
- whole grains (rich in magnesium);
- nuts and grains (rich in magnesium);
- vegetable protein, as in tofu.

Choose a diet low in:

- saturated fat and cholesterol;
- sodium: a moderate amount of sodium a day – approximately 2300 mg or 1 teaspoon (5 ml) of salt – is recommended for people with diabetes.

The main sources of sodium are processed foods (77%), naturally occurring sodium (12%), salt added at the table (6%), and salt added in cooking (5%).

Choosing fresh food over processed (e.g., sauces, condiments, soups, frozen or ready-to-serve meals) can greatly reduce sodium consumption.

- Buy unsalted or low-sodium foods. Look for "sodium free," "low sodium" or "unsalted" on the packaging.
- Look for food containing less than 360 mg of sodium per portion.

- Check the percent daily value (% DV) on the label to compare products and determine whether the sodium content of the food is high or low.
- Choose products containing less than 15% of your daily value of sodium.

Use the "Sodium Detector" tool in the "Health Risks of Too Much Sodium" section of Health Canada's website to find out how much sodium is hiding in some foods.[5]

If you drink alcohol, moderate amounts can help control blood pressure. Follow the low-risk alcohol-consumption guidelines in "National Alcohol Strategy: Reducing Alcohol-Related Harm in Canada." Healthy adults should limit their alcohol consumption to:

- 1–10 standard glasses a week for women; at most, 3 glasses a day, most days of the week.
- 0–15 standard glasses a week for men; at most 4 glasses a day, most days of the week.

See chapter 11 for more details on the size of a standard glass, depending on the type of alcohol.

Some people with diabetes, however – particularly those who take medications putting them at risk of hypoglycemia (e.g., insulin or Diaßeta®) – are advised to have a snack containing carbohydrates (approximately 15 g) in the evening, as late as possible before going to bed. It is preferable for the snack to contain a protein source such as milk (e.g. 125 mL or ½ cup milk and 2 dry biscuits).

Can a person with diabetes still enjoy eating?

Getting the most out of eating means involving all of your senses, from meal planning, through preparation, to the final enjoyment of the food.

Taking the time to consult interesting cookbooks, choosing the recipes, and planning a creative meal are all ways of enhancing the pleasure of eating.

Markets display an array of colourful and aromatic foods and can present an opportunity to discuss flavours, aromas, and recipes with other food lovers. Preparing meals alone or with others can be a simple task but still provide a chance to experiment with a variety of new flavours and sensations. Attractive food presentation and an inviting table add to the satisfaction of a delicious and healthy meal.

What are some ways to develop better nutritional habits?

Here are some suggestions:

- First, set clear, measurable, and realistic goals.
- Go about it gradually, one change at a time. Small adjustments can make a big difference.
- See a dietitian specialized in diabetes.
- Be sure that you like the food you choose; being satisfied is the best way to prevent slips.
- Replace food rewards with other treats. For example, buy a book, go for a walk in the country, or take a relaxing bath to pamper yourself.

---

5 http://www.hc-sc.gc.ca/hl-vs/iyh-vsv/food-aliment/sodium-eng.php

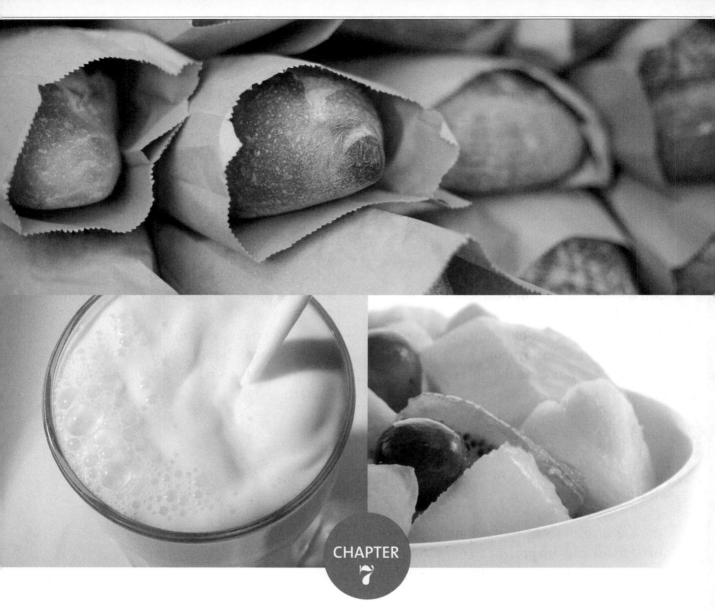

Getting to Know Carbohydrates

What are dietary carbohydrates?

Dietary carbohydrates, which are stored in the liver and muscles after digestion, are used by the body as fuel. Although they have an effect on blood glucose levels, foods containing carbohydrates are a vital part of every meal.

PRIMARY DIETARY CARBOHYDRATES	SOURCES
Glucose (also known as dextrose)	• glucose tablets (also used by the nutrition industry)
Sucrose (saccharose)	• table sugar
Fructose	• fruit • honey • agave syrup
Lactose	• dairy products
Starch	• cereal • legumes • tubers • root vegetables • some types of fruit
Dietary fibre	• whole grain products • fruit • vegetables • legumes • nuts and seeds • wheat and oat bran
Polyols (sugar alcohols)	• used as sugar substitutes

What are the most common approaches to integrating carbohydrates into meals?

THE EXCHANGE SYSTEM

This system involves grouping foods according to their nutritional content (protein, carbohydrates and fats). All the foods in the same group have the same nutritional content, and single portions of food within the same group are known as exchanges.

Foods within the same group are interchangeable, so long as the same number of exchanges per meal is consumed. Exchanges between the starches, fruit, and milk and milk alternatives groups are also possible, provided the diet remains varied.

This system categorizes food into seven main groups:

- Starches
- Fruit
- Vegetables
- Milk and alternatives
- Other foods
- Meat and alternatives
- Fats

An eighth group of "low-calorie foods" has recently been added. There are no restrictions on the consumption of foods in this group, given their negligible effect on blood glucose and blood lipids.

Each exchange contains on average 15 g of carbohydrates or 3 teaspoons of sugar, except for vegetables, meat, and fats. One exchange of vegetables contains an average of 5 g of carbohydrates or 1 teaspoon of sugar. Most raw and cooked vegetables contain few carbohydrates and therefore have little effect on blood glucose. Vegetables with the highest carbohydrate content are included in the starches group, which have an effect on blood glucose.

The exchange system is used primarily to plan meals for people with diabetes whose treatment consists of diet, antidiabetic medications, or fixed-dose insulin therapy.

It is used by Diabetes Québec (DQ), who provides a detailed explanation the brochures entitled *Meal Planning for People with Diabetes*[1] and *A Glance at Meal Planning for People with Diabetes*.[2] It is also used by the American Diabetes Association (ADA). The system recommended by the Canadian Diabetes Association (CDA), which has recently been revised, closely resembles the one used by Diabetes Québec and the ADA, and is outlined in a simplified guide entitled *Just the Basics: Tips for Healthy Eating, Diabetes Prevention and Management*.[3]

The table opposite lists the exchange systems, the differences between them, and a few examples of exchanges.

In a meal, when a food portion contains less than **3 g of carbohydrates** and only one portion is consumed, these carbohydrates should not be included in the total carbohydrate count of the meal.

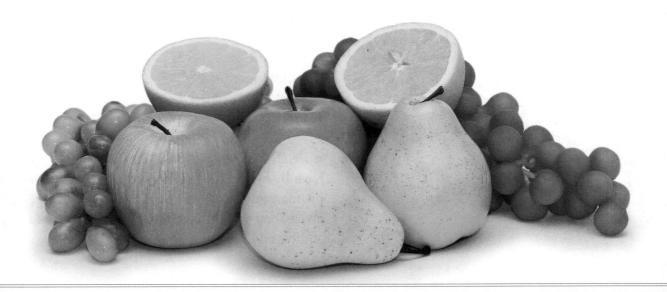

AMOUNT OF CARBOHYDRATES IN AN EXCHANGE			
Food groups	Systems		ONE SERVING CORRESPONDING TO ONE EXCHANGE
DQ/CDA	DQ and ADA	CDA	
Starches/Grains and starches	15 g	15 g	• 1 slice of bread weighing 30 g • 75 mL (⅓ cup) of pasta • 25 mL (½ cup) of lentils • 250 mL (1 cup) of green peas
Fruit	15 g	15 g	• ½ banana • 2 small kiwis • 125 mL (½ cup) orange juice
Vegetables	0 g to 5 g	–	• 125 mL (½ cup) fresh, frozen or canned vegetables • 250 mL (1 cup) leafy raw vegetables
Milk and alternatives/ Dairy products and alternatives	12 g to 15 g	15 g	• 250 mL (1 cup) of milk • 175 mL (¾ cup) of plain yogurt
Other foods	15 g	15 g	• 125 mL (½ cup) flavoured gelatin (Jell-O®)
Meat and alternatives	0 g	0 g	• 30 g or 1 ounce of chicken, meat or fish
Fats	0 g	0 g	• 5 mL (1 tsp) oil, margarine or butter
Low-calorie foods/ Extras	< 5 g	< 5 g	• Spices, diet drinks

BASIC CARBOHYDRATE COUNTING

This method involves planning how many grams of carbohydrates will be in each meal and snack. Basic carbohydrate counting can be used by anyone with diabetes and is especially useful for people who have trouble using the food exchange system.

ADVANCED CARBOHYDRATE COUNTING

Advanced carbohydrate counting involves counting the total carbohydrates of every meal as precisely as possible. This method is particularly useful for people with diabetes who inject insulin for a variable carbohydrate diet.

1 http://publications.msss.gouv.qc.ca/acrobat/f/ documentation/2010/10-215-02FA.pdf or by telephone at 514 644-4545 or toll-free at 1 877 644-4545
2 http://publications.msss.gouv.qc.ca/acrobat/f/ documentation/2009/09-215-01F.pdf
3 http://www.diabetes.ca/files/JTB17x_11_CPGO3_1103.pdf or by telephone at 1 800 BANTING.

The amount of insulin for each meal is calculated using an insulin-to-carbohydrate ratio (that is, a certain number of units of insulin for every 10 g of carbohydrates). The insulin dose is thus proportionate to the amount of carbohydrates consumed. Initially, the doctor determines the insulin-to-carbohydrate ratio for the specific person, although it can also be determined by using a dietary journal recording the amount of carbohydrates consumed at every meal, the amount of insulin injected, and blood glucose readings. Ratios may differ from one meal to another over the course of the same day.

Advanced carbohydrate counting allows for a certain amount of flexibility, since it does not require planning the specific amount of carbohydrates for every meal and snack.

Where can information on the carbohydrate content of specific foods be found?

There are a number of ways to learn the carbohydrate content of foods.

Product labels

A nutrition facts label is printed on pre-packaged food products. It lists the total amount of carbohydrates in grams of a specified portion of that food. Sugars, dietary fibre, starches and polyols (sugar alcohols) are included in the carbohydrate count.

- The term "sugars" designates carbohydrates like glucose, fructose, sucrose (saccharose), and lactose. They may occur naturally or be added to the food.
- Polyols (alcohol sugars) refer to carbohydrates such as maltitol, mannitol, and sorbitol.

Food composition tables

Health Canada publishes a useful food composition table entitled *Nutrient Value of Some Common Foods* (2008).

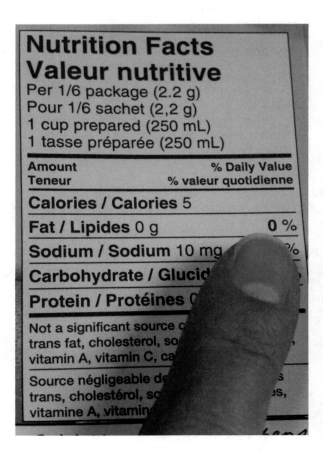

Nutritional information provided by restaurants

Some restaurants provide nutritional information about the food they serve. Be sure to ask.

Cookbooks

Some cookbooks provide a nutritional breakdown of the recipes.

Lists of exchanges

A dietitian-nutritionist can provide lists of food exchanges. You can also refer to lists published by the Ministère de la Santé et des Services sociaux and Diabetes Québec (*Meal Planning for People with Diabetes*) and by the Canadian Diabetes Association (*Just the Basics: Meal Planning for Eating, Diabetes Prevention and Management*).

Carbohydrate factors

The carbohydrate factor is the amount of carbohydrates in 1 g of a given food. For example:

- one 100 g pear with a carbohydrate factor of 0.12 contains 12 g total carbohydrates:
  100 g x 0.12 = 12 g of carbohydrates

A table of carbohydrate factors can be found in the book *Pumping Insulin*.

What amount of carbohydrates should be eaten daily?

Total daily carbohydrate intake is determined by energy (or caloric) needs, which are evaluated according to a person's size, weight, sex, age and level of physical activity. A minimum of 130 g should be consumed daily to provide the brain with the energy it needs to function.

In a balanced diet, carbohydrates should provide on average half of a person's caloric needs. The rest should be supplied by proteins and fats.

Generally, for an adult, the amount should fall between 200 g and 300 g per day. This corresponds to:

- 45 g to 60 g of carbohydrates per meal for women;
- 60 g to 75 g of carbohydrates per meal for men.

4 http://www.hc-sc.gc.ca/fn-an/alt_formats/pdf/nutrition/fiche-nutri-data/nvscf-vnqau-eng.pdf (to order this booklet over the telephone, see chapter 28).
5 John Walsh & Ruth Roberts, *Pumping Insulin*, 4th ed.
(Torrey Pines Press, 2006).

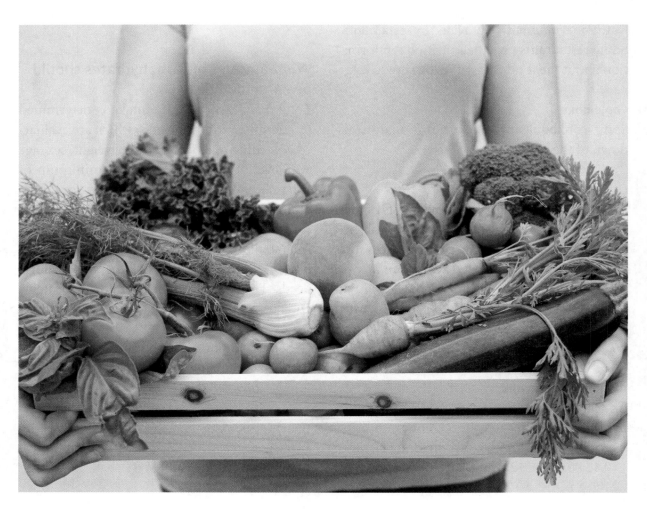

What is the impact of different types of carbohydrates on diabetes?

Added sugar: The American Heart Association and the World Health Organization recently recommended limiting the amount of added sugar to a maximum of 5 to 9 teaspoons a day, depending on the number of calories ingested, to prevent diabetes and obesity. The subject is currently a matter of some debate.

Sugar should be consumed only occasionally because sugar-rich foods often contain many calories and are usually low in nutrients. The most important thing to remember is that added sugar is not toxic, and when consumed on its own or in food it must be counted as part of the carbohydrate content of the meal.

Fibre: A variety of fibre-rich foods are advised. A good source of vitamins and minerals, fibre does not increase blood glucose because it resists digestion by human enzymes in the small intestine and thus is fermented in the large bowel.

Fibre should be introduced gradually to avoid unpleasant effects such as bloating and flatulence. It is also important to drink a sufficient amount of liquid to help fibre perform its role efficiently.

It has been shown that, for people with diabetes, soluble fibre such as that found in eggplant, oats, legumes, okra, barley and psyllium slow down digestion and delay the absorption of glucose in the intestine, thus improving postprandial blood glucose levels. Moreover, diets rich in fibre from grains are associated with a decrease in the risk of cardiovascular disease.

For all of these reasons, the amount of fibre suggested for people with diabetes is between 25 g and 50 g a day, which is higher than the recommendation for the general population.

Dietary fibre has a number of other benefits. For example:

- Fibre fights constipation: Fibre improves intestinal transit, increases the volume of stool, and helps the large intestine (colon) perform better.
- Fibre positively affects blood cholesterol: Large amounts of fibre can help lower blood cholesterol.
- Fibre helps weight control: Foods rich in fibre cause a feeling of fullness and are lower in calories.

Fructose: Some studies have shown that when the carbohydrates in a meal are replaced by the same amount of fructose, the added fructose does not have a harmful effect on the weight or blood pressure of people with diabetes, and could even have a positive effect on blood glucose levels. However, eating more than 60 g a day can cause a slight increase in blood triglycerides (a type of fat in the blood) and could contribute to weight gain.

The consumption of fructose in fruit has no harmful effect on people with diabetes so long as the fruit is eaten in small quantities, following the suggestions in "Eating Well with Canada's Food Guide," which advises 7 to 10 portions of fruit and vegetables. Choosing fruit with a low glycemic index can further improve blood glucose levels.

Should the same amount of carbohydrates be eaten every day?

It depends on the person's treatment regimen.

- **People with diabetes whose treatment consists solely of diet or of diet combined with fixed medical treatment** (either oral antidiabetic drugs or insulin) should eat the same amount of carbohydrates at every meal and have a regular meal schedule.

The total amount of carbohydrates should be spread out over the course of the day. This will help avoid a spike in blood glucose after meals.

- **People who count carbohydrates and inject insulin according to the amount of carbohydrates ingested** may vary their carbohydrate consumption from one day to another.

Whatever the type of treatment, balanced meals should remain a priority, as they are vital to good health. Overeating or nutritional imbalance can lead to weight gain and the development of health problems such as high blood pressure or high cholesterol.

What is the glycemic index?

According to the CDA, the glycemic index is a scale ranking carbohydrate-rich foods by their ability to raise blood glucose levels after consumption, compared to a reference food, either glucose or white bread. Low glycemic index foods (e.g. legumes) cause blood glucose to rise more gradually than high glycemic index foods (e.g., white bread or mashed potatoes).

Here are some foods that rank low on the glycemic index:
- milled or stone ground whole grains
- oatmeal
- legumes
- sweet potatoes
- pasta
- barley

It is now recognized that taking the glycemic index of food into account when planning meals makes carbohydrate counting even more effective. Low glycemic index foods are said to help control blood glucose levels after meals, although studies are contradictory. It nevertheless seems clear that low glycemic index foods, especially those high in fibre, positively influence insulin sensitivity and even the pancreatic insulin secretion.[6]

6 http://www.diabetes.ca/files/glycemicindex_08.pdf

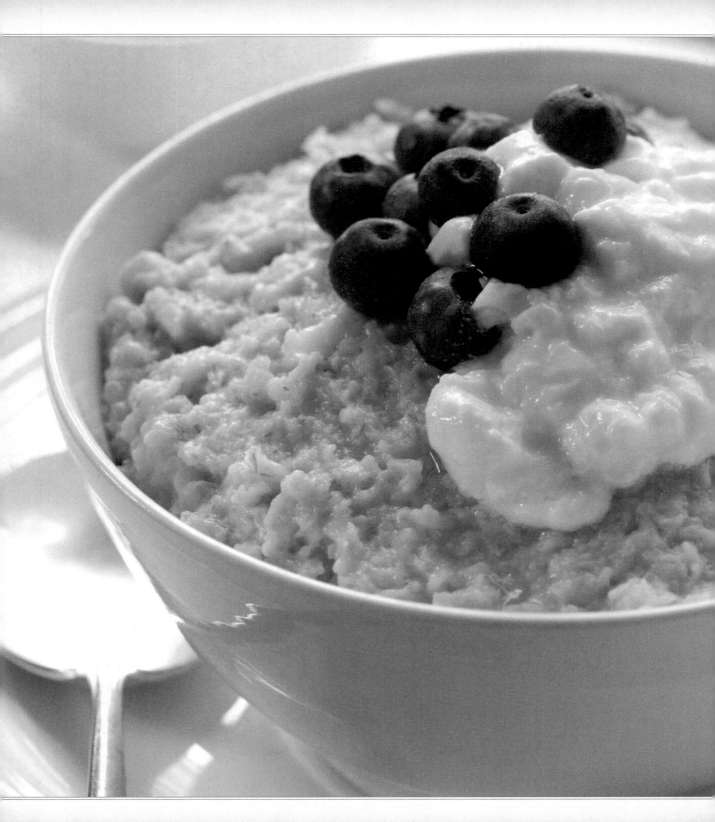

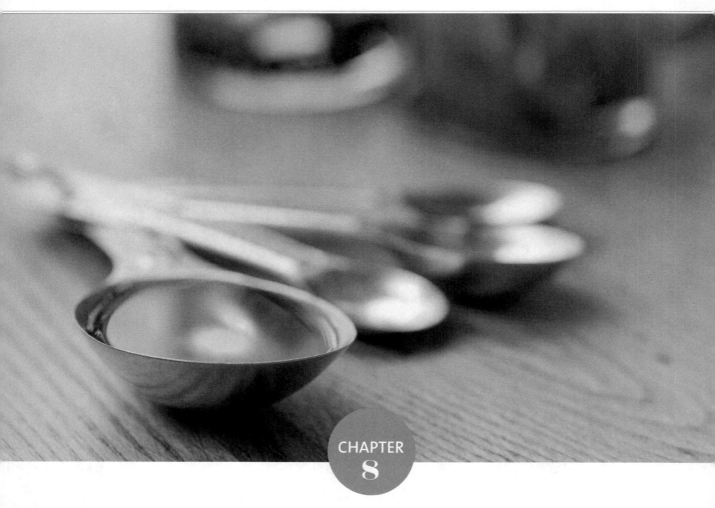

Fats:
Making the Right Choices

What types of fats occur naturally in foods?

The following types of fats occur naturally:

- saturated fats, usually of animal origin;
- cholesterol, always of animal origin;
- unsaturated fats, primarily from plants (monounsaturated and polyunsaturated);
- trans fats, naturally present in small quantities in meats and dairy products.

Foods are classified according to their predominant fat source, as no food contains only one type of fat.

Sunflower oil, for example, contains small amounts of saturated and monounsaturated fat, but it is very high in polyunsaturated fats. It is therefore classified as a source of polyunsaturated fat.

Visible fats	Invisible fats
• Oil • Butter • Margarine • Lard • Tallow or beef fat • Vegetable oil • Meats	• Meats and cold cuts • Fatty fish (e.g., mackerel and herring) • Sauces (e.g., mayonnaise, béarnaise, white or cheese) • Some types of prepared dishes • Cookies, pastries, croissants, brioche • Avocados • Olives • Fried food and chips • 8-10% M.F. yogurt • Cheese • Cream • Nuts and seeds

Which foods contain fats?

The following foods contain either visible or hidden fat:

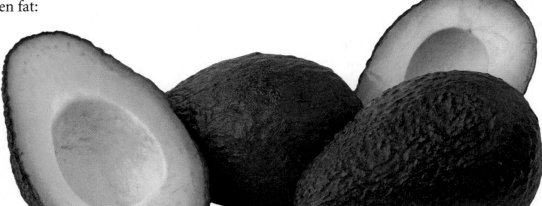

Why do fats need to be chosen carefully?

When a person has diabetes, the risk of developing cardiovascular disease is elevated. If the level of triglycerides and bad cholesterol are too high in the blood, the risk increases even more.

To prevent cardiovascular disease, choose fats carefully and limit the amount you eat. This has the added benefit of preventing weight gain or obesity.

For people at risk of developing cardiovascular disease, the different types of fats and the foods that contain them can have either negative or positive effects on the level of fats in the blood (blood lipids), which are:

- triglycerides;
- total cholesterol;
- HDL cholesterol (good cholesterol);
- LDL cholesterol (bad cholesterol).

Because of their healthful effects, foods containing monounsaturated and polyunsaturated fats should be preferred to those containing saturated fats, trans or hydrogenated fats, or cholesterol.

Foods containing **monounsaturated and polyunsaturated** fats include oils, dehydrogenated margarine, fatty fish, nuts and seeds, avocados, olives, and any food made with these fat sources.

The following table lists the main foods recognized as sources of mono- and polyunsaturated fats.

SOURCES OF UNSATURATED FATS	
monounsaturated	polyunsaturated
• Almonds	• Pumpkin seeds
• Peanuts	• Flax seeds
• Avocados	• Sunflower seeds
• Sesame seeds	• Borage oil
• Peanut oil	• Safflower oil
• Canola oil	• Pumpkin oil
• Hazelnut oil	• Flax oil
• Sesame oil	• Corn oil
• Olive oil	• Nut oil
• Hazelnuts	• Grapeseed oil
• Cashews	• Soya oil
• Brazil nuts	• Sunflower oil
• Olives	• Evening primrose oil
• Pecans	• Walnuts
• Pistachios	• Pine nuts
	• Fatty fish (salmon, mackerel, etc.)

SOURCES OF UNSATURATED FATS
monounsaturated and polyunsaturated
Soft, dehydrogenated margarines (e.g., Becel®, Crystal®, Lactantia®, Nuvel®, Olivina®, etc.)

If fats can be bad for me, why do I have to eat them?

Fats are part of a balanced diet, just like carbohydrates and proteins. They are an excellent source of energy. They contain essential fatty acids, which help make up certain vitamins and hormones, and play a vital role in the body.

Which foods are known to be sources of saturated and trans fat?

SOURCES OF TRANS OR HYDROGENATED FATS
Plant origin
• Partially hydrogenated vegetable oil • Partially hydrogenated soft margarine • Hard margarine • Vegetable shortening • Some bakery products • Fast food • Fried snacks • Non-dairy creamers (e.g., CoffeeMate®)

SOURCES OF SATURATED FATS
Animal origin*
• Butter • Cream, ice cream • Cheese • Whole milk (3.25% M.F.) • Lard • Eggs • Tallow or beef fat • Meat • Poultry and skin • Yogurt 8% M.F.
Plant origin
• Coconut or copra oil • Palm oil • Palm kernel oil • Coconut

* These foods also contain cholesterol.

What do I need to know about hydrogenated and trans fats?

Small amounts of trans fats occur naturally in certain foods, including dairy products, beef, and lamb. They can also form when oils are industrially processed from a liquid to a solid state. Partially hydrogenated margarine, vegetable fats, and fats used for certain bakery products are a few examples.

Regular consumption of hydrogenated or trans fats, just like saturated fats, increases the risk of cardiovascular disease. Only limited amounts should be eaten. Always look at the nutrition facts label on food packaging to choose products containing little or no trans fat.

In June 2007, Health Canada adopted the recommendations of a working group seeking to reduce the trans fat content of foods and gave the food industry two years to ensure that trans fat content was limited to:

- 2% of the total amount of fats in oils and soft margarine;
- 5% of the total in other foods, including ingredients sold or prepared in restaurants.

The Trans Fat Monitoring Program analyzed a vast range of foods and provided data on restaurants, fast-food establishments, ethnic food establishments, as well as nutritional information. The monitoring program came to an end in 2009 but may continue to monitor certain food groups.

Why does fat consumption lead to weight gain?

One gram of carbohydrates or protein contains four calories. One gram of fat, on the other hand, contains nine calories, more than double.

- 5 mL or 1 teaspoon of sugar (5 g of carbohydrates) contains 20 calories;
- 5 mL or 1 teaspoon of oil (5 g of fat) contains about 45 calories.

Should people with diabetes count fats the way they count carbohydrates?

Not necessarily. In most cases, there are other ways (eating smaller portions of meat or choosing lower-fat cheeses, for example) to reduce the amount of dietary fat to a satisfactory level. People usually eat large quantities of fat on impulse because it adds flavour, making the food more appealing.

How can the consumption of fats — trans or hydrogenated fats in particular — be reduced?

Remember that:

- all fats have comparable energy value: 5 mL or 1 teaspoon of oil, butter, or margarine all contain 40 to 45 calories;
- no oil is low-fat; the term "light" to describe oils refers to the taste.

To eat less fat, do the following:

- Develop the habit of measuring fats with a teaspoon or tablespoon: one teaspoon equals 5 mL and one tablespoon equals 15 mL.[1]
- Choose leaner cuts of meat (10% or less fat), poultry, fish, molluscs, and crustaceans on occasion; trim visible fat and remove skin before cooking.
- Eat reasonably sized servings of meat or alternatives, no bigger than the palm of your hand; a meat serving that size equals 90 g (3 oz) of meat.
- Eat fish more often, at least two or three times a week.
- Incorporate legumes (beans, etc.) into your meals.
- Eat less cheese or select leaner cheeses more often; leaner choices include unripened cheeses (for example, cottage, quark, goat milk, bocconcini). Cheese with over 20% fat content has two or three times more fat than meat.

- Drink partially skimmed or skimmed milk (1% M.F. or 2% M.F.) instead of whole milk (3.25% M.F.).
- Reduce daily consumption of fatty foods like butter and cream sauces, pastries, pre-packaged muffins, croissants, brioches, cookies, and so on. Save these foods for special occasions only. Replace them with yogurt, mousses, desserts made with skimmed or partially skimmed milk, puddings, soy mousses, dry cookies, homemade muffins and dessert breads, etc.

---

1 1 soup spoon equals 1 tablespoon or 3 teaspoons.

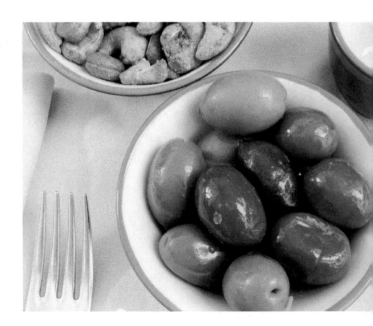

Which cooking methods can result in lower fat content?

When cooking, use methods requiring the least amount of fat possible. The following table provides examples of low-fat cooking methods and some suggested dishes.

Cooking method	Dishes
Water	Boiled beef, boiled chicken
Steam	Vegetables, fish, pressure-cooked or steamed rice
Conventional or microwave oven	Poultry, roasts (beef, chicken, veal), fish, fruit, gratin with light béchamel
Double-boiler	Scrambled eggs
Braising	Mixed dishes cooked in a clay pot or pressure cooker
Grill	Cast-iron, oven or BBQ grill: meats, poultry, vegetables, higher-fat fish such as salmon
Frying	Non-stick frying pan for eggs, omelettes and sliced meat
Closed packet (papillote)	Fish, lean meats, potatoes, fruits
Simmered or stewed	Stewing meats
Gros sel*	Fish, chicken

* Heat the gros sel (coarse sea salt) in the oven between two aluminum plates for approximately 30 minutes at 500°F (260°C). Remove from the oven and place the chicken or fish in the salt. Cook 30 minutes at 350°F (175°C).

Can some foods help lower blood fat levels?

Vegetable sterols (phytosterols), soy proteins (with isoflavones), soluble fibre, and nuts can reduce cholesterol. Some diets can have the same effect. Marine omega-3 fatty acids help lower triglyceride levels. The following table displays the expected benefits of certain changes in diet and lifestyle and the minimum change required.

Change in diet	Benefit
Reduce cholesterol (less than 300 mg per day)	▼ LDL
Reduce saturated fat (less than 7% of total calories)	▼ LDL ▼ cardiovascular death
Add 1 to 2 g of phytosterols per day	▼ LDL
Add 25 g of soy protein (with isoflavones) per day	▼ LDL
Add 10 g of soluble fibre per day	▼ LDL
Add 30 g of nuts per day	▼ LDL and ▼ TG
Add 2 to 4 g of omega-3 per day	▼ TG
Lose 5% to 10% of current weight and reduce waist size	▼ LDL ▲ HDL ▼ TG
Mediterranean diet	▼ LDL ▲ HDL ▼ TG ▼ cardiovascular death
Vegetarian diet	▼ LDL and ▲ HDL
DASH diet	▼ LDL and ▲ HDL
Diet rich in legumes	▼ LDL
Change in lifestyle	Benefit
30 to 60 minutes of moderate to intense exercise a day	▲ HDL ▼ cardiovascular events
1 to 2 (moderate) alcoholic drinks a day	▲ HDL
Quit smoking	▲ HDL ▼ cardiovascular events

Adapted from Anderson, et al., Can U. Cardiol. 2012; 29:151–167 and CDA Clinical Practice Guidelines 2013, Chapter 11: *Nutrition Therapy*.

▼ decreaser ▲ increase

Vegetable sterols (phytosterols) have a beneficial effect on LDL-cholesterol (bad cholesterol). They partially block the absorption of cholesterol in the intestine, thereby reducing the amount of bad cholesterol in the blood. The recommended daily consumption is approximately 2 grams of vegetable sterols. They occur naturally in vegetable oils, nuts, seeds, and whole grains, but only in very small quantities. Because huge quantities of these foods would have to be consumed in order to have any effect, sterols are marketed as supplements and added to certain foods, including certain types of margarine (e.g., Becel®, pro.activ® and Oasis Health Break CholestPrevent® orange juice).

Soluble fibre also has a beneficial effect on bad cholesterol, especially for people with high cholesterol. The recommended daily consumption is 10 g. Spreading it out over three meals also maximizes its beneficial effect on postprandial blood glucose.

The following foods contain approximately 3 g of soluble fibre per portion

Food	Portion
All-Bran Buds® cereal	75 mL (⅓ cup)
Canned artichoke hearts	2
Ground flax seed	60 mL (¼ cup)
Roasted soy seeds	60 mL (¼ cup)
Uncooked oatmeal	175 mL (¾ cup)
Cooked red beans	125 mL (½ cup)
Metamucil®	15 mL (1 tbsp.)
Fresh pear	1
Psyllium powder or flakes	10 mL (2 tsp.)
Uncooked oat bran	100 mL (7 tbsp.)

From Chantal Blais et al., "Dyslipidémie" (chapter) in D. Decelles, M. Daignault Gélinas, L. Lavallée Côté et al., *Manuel de nutrition clinique en ligne*, (Montreal: Ordre professionnel des diététistes du Québec, 2006).

Marine omega-3 fatty acids have documented effects on triglycerides. The general population is advised to eat fish one to three times a week. It is better to eat fish than to take omega-3 supplements.

The following table provides a few examples of the best nutritional sources of marine omega-3 fatty acids.

Food 75 g (2 ½ oz) portion	Total amount of omega-3 (g)
Atlantic herring, smoked and salted	1.72
Cooked Atlantic salmon	1.7
Atlantic herring, baked or grilled	1.61
Canned pink (sockeye) salmon, drained, with skin and bones, salted	1.46
Fresh red tuna, baked or grilled	1.13
Atlantic sardines in oil, drained, with bones	1.11
Blue mackerel, baked or grilled	0.99
Canned keta (chum) salmon, drained, with skin and bones, salted	0.93
Wild or farmed rainbow trout, cooked	0.93
Canned pink salmon, drained, with skin and bones, salted	0.84
Canned white tuna, in water	0.70

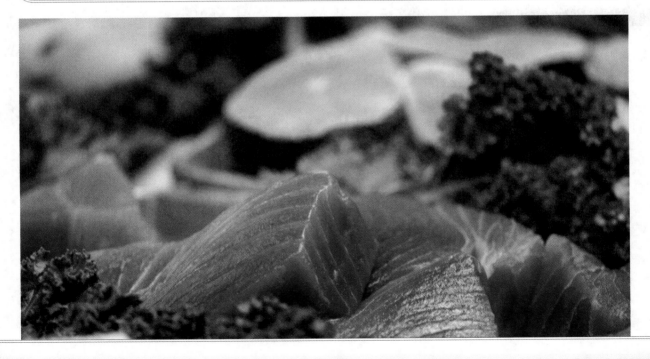

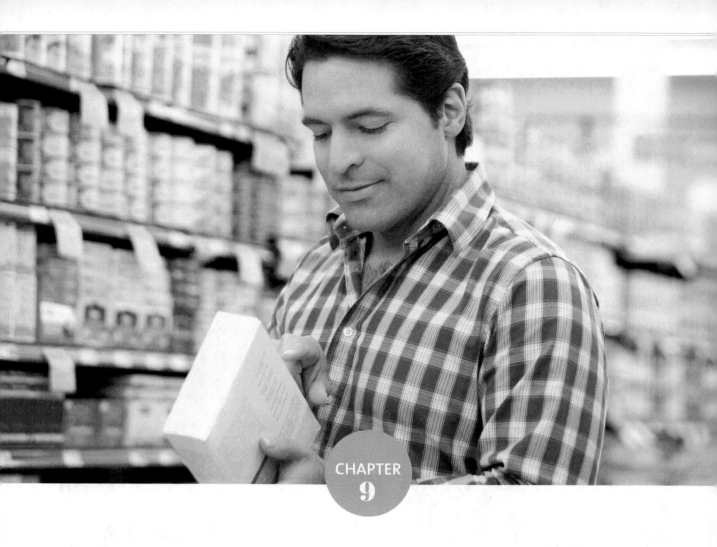

How to Read Food Labels

What information is listed on prepackaged food labels?

The food labels on prepackaged food contains the following nutritional information:

- the Nutrition Facts table;
- the list of ingredients;
- the product's nutritional and health claims.

Health Canada regulates food labelling in Canada through the *Food and Drugs Act*. The regulation governing labelling has been updated and its latest version was published on January 1, 2003. Since December 2007, nutritional labelling has been mandatory on all prepackaged foods.

The Canadian Food Inspection Agency (CFIA) is responsible for protecting the public against fraud or misrepresentation.[1]

What information is listed in the Nutrition Facts table?

The Nutrition Facts table on prepackaged food labels provides information about a specified quantity of the food. This information includes:

- the caloric value of the food in the specified serving;
- the content of 13 listed nutrients in the specified serving;
- the percentage of the recommended daily value (% DV) represented by that serving.

NUTRITION FACTS per 125 mL (87 g)	
Amount	% Daily Value
Calories 80	
Fat 0.5 g	1%
Saturated 0g	
+trans	
Cholesterol 0 mg	
Sodium 0 mg	0%
Carbohydrates 18 g	6 %
Fibre 2 g	
Sugars 2 g	
Protein 3 g	
Vitamin A 2%	Vitamin C 10%
Calcium 0%	Iron 2%

In the Nutrition Facts label, the percentage of the daily value (% DV) can help you make an informed choice when comparing two similar food products. Remember the following:

- 5% DV or less is little;
- 15% or more is a lot.

The % DV can be used to help you choose foods with either more or less nutritional value.

For example:
If you want to decrease your sodium intake, choose foods with a low % DV of sodium.
If you want to increase your fibre intake, choose foods with a higher % DV of fibre.

---

1 See the following web sites on food labelling in Canada: http://www.hc-sc.gc.ca/fn-an/label-etiquet/nutrition/index-eng.php; http://www.hc-sc.gc.ca/fn-an/label-etiquet/index-eng.php

What information is in the list of ingredients?

The list includes all of the food's ingredients, presented in decreasing order of weight; in other words, the ingredients present in the greatest amount are listed first.

What should I know about the manufacturer's nutritional claims?

The nutrition labelling regulation permits two types of nutritional claims:

- **Nutrient content claims**, which are statements or expressions describing the nutritional elements of a food.
- **Health claims**, which include any representation affirming, suggesting or implying a relationship between a food or an ingredient in the food and a health effect.

Nutrient content and health claims are useful for people with diabetes as they can help them make better-informed nutritional choices.

What are some nutrient content claims that appear on labels?

The following chart presents several examples of nutrient content claims on food product labels, along with their meanings.

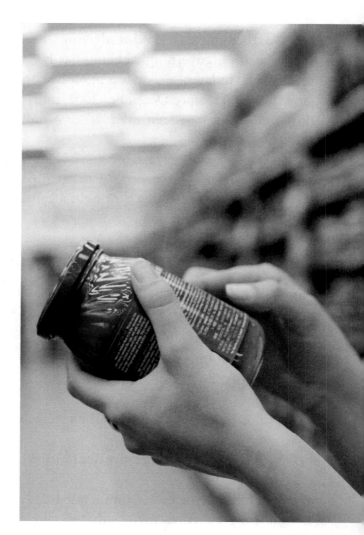

CLAIMS	MEANING PER COMPARED OR SPECIFIED SERVING
Energy*	
"Calorie-reduced"	At least 25% lower in calories than the similar food to which it is compared
"Low-calorie"	No more than 40 calories
"Calorie-free"	Less than 5 calories
Lipids**	
"Fat free"	Less than 0.5 g of fat
"Low fat"	No more than 3 g of fat
"Low in saturated fat"	No more than 2 g of saturated fat and trans fat in total, and no more than 15% of total calories derived from saturated fat and trans fat
"No trans fatty acids"	Less than 0.2 g of trans fatty acids and "low in saturated fat"
Cholesterol	
"Cholesterol free"	Less than 2 mg of cholesterol and low in saturated fat
Carbohydrates and sugar	
"Sugar free"	Less than 0.5 g of sugar
"Reduced sugar"	At least 25% less sugar than the similar food to which it is compared
"No added sugar"	No added sugar such as saccharose, fructose, glucose, molasses, fruit juice, honey, syrup, etc
Fibre	
"Source of fibre"	2 g or more of fibre
"Good source of fibre"	4 g or more of fibre
"Very good source of fibre"	6 g or more of fibre
Calcium	
"Good source of calcium"	At least 165 mg of calcium

* "Energy" can be replaced by "Calories"
** "Lipids" can be replaced by "Fats"

When the term "light" appears on a product, the manufacturer must indicate the justification for this claim on the label. When the term "light" refers to its nutritional value, the term is authorized only for food low in calories or low in fat.

What kinds of health claims are authorized?

Manufacturers may include diet claims on a food product, provided that the claim is based on scientifically demonstrated links between the food product and a reduced risk of chronic disease, such as the following:

- A low-sodium and high-potassium diet may reduce the risk of high blood pressure.
- A healthy diet with adequate calcium and vitamin D may reduce the risk of osteoporosis.
- A diet low in saturated and trans fats may reduce the risk of cardiovascular disease.
- A diet rich in fruits and vegetables may reduce the risk of certain types of cancer.

A permitted health claim, for example, could read as follows:
"A healthy diet including a variety of fruits and vegetables may help reduce the risk of certain types of cancer."

How is the law applied?

The Canadian Food Inspection Agency (CFIA)[2] is in charge of implementing inspections to determine whether nutritional information is in compliance with the regulations the government enacted in 2003.

What is a sugar substitute?

A sugar substitute is a substance that replaces table sugar (saccharose or sucrose) as a food sweetener. Some add calories or carbohydrates and are known as nutritive sweeteners; others do not and are therefore called non-nutritive. Any calories or carbohydrates added by nutritive sweeteners will have some effect on blood glucose levels so they must be included in the carbohydrate count or meal plan. Non-nutritive sweeteners have no calories and little effect on blood glucose.

What types of nutritive sugar substitutes can be found in prepackaged foods?

The following chart presents the various nutritive sugar substitutes that increase blood glucose, along with a few of their properties.

In the above table, the sugar substitutes ending with "-ol" as well as hydrogenated starch hydrolysate are known collectively as "polyols" or "sugar alcohols." They come from fruit plants or berries, but they can also be synthetically manufactured.

Compared to table sugar (sucrose), sugar alcohols provide fewer calories and carbohydrates and have less of an effect on blood glucose because they are digested more slowly or only partially absorbed by the intestine. Foods containing nutritive sugar substitutes include gum, candy, chocolate, jam, ice cream, syrup, nutrition bars, and cough drops.

Nutritive sweeteners	Some properties
Fructose	• Possible effect on blood glucose, triglycerides, cholesterol and weight • Consumption of more than 60 g per day is not recommended for people with diabetes • Risk of gastro-intestinal symptoms
Sorbitol Mannitol Xylitol Isomalt Maltitol Hydrogenated starch hydrolysate	• Provides fewer calories than sugars because they are only partly absorbed • Glycemic response is weaker than sugars • Do not cause cavities • Risk of gastro-intestinal symptoms due to varying degrees of laxative effect
Lactitol	• Not absorbed; provides calories • No glycemic effect • Risk of gastro-intestinal symptoms due to varying degrees of laxative effect

---

2 http://www.inspection.gc.ca

What non-nutritive sugar substitutes are authorized in Canada and are found in some prepackaged foods?

The following chart lists some non-nutritive sugar substitutes that do not increase blood glucose, along with some general information about them.

The permissible daily dose in this table is the estimated safe dose if the sugar substitute is consumed every day over a lifetime

Other sugar substitutes approved by Health Canada – specifically, neotame, thaumatin, erythritol, and D-tagatose – can be found on ingredient lists on prepackaged foods.

Non-nutritive sugar substitute	Brand names	Sources	ADI* mg/kg/day	Daily maximum** (mg)
Acesulfame potassium	Not on the market	• Prepackaged foods or drinks	15	750
Aspartame	• Equal® • NutraSweet® • Sweet'N'Low® • Private brands	• Packets, tablets or powder • Prepackaged foods or drinks	40	2000
Cyclamates	• Sucaryl® • SugarTwin® • Sweet'N'Low® • Private brands	• Packets, tablets, powder or liquid • Unauthorized in prepackaged foods or drinks	11***	550
Saccharine	Hermesetas®	• Packets, tablets • Unauthorized in prepackaged foods or drinks	5***	250
Sucralose	Splenda®	• Packets, tablets • Prepackaged foods or drinks	9	450
Steviol glycosides	Stevia	• Prepackaged foods or drinks	4	200

* ADI = Acceptable Daily Intake.
** For a 50-kg (110 lb) adult
*** Not recommended during pregnancy or while breastfeeding

In 2012, Health Canada approved the use of purified stevia (steviol glycoside) extracts as a food additive, table sweetener, and sweetener for some categories of foods.

The stevia leaf and its raw extracts are considered to be food ingredients, not food additives, and have been approved by Health Canada as non-medicinal ingredients in certain natural health products.

How are sugar alcohols listed in the Nutrition Facts table on prepackaged foods?

They are listed under total carbohydrates and frequently referred to as "sugar alcohols" or by their specific names.

How are carbohydrates that potentially affect blood glucose measured in products containing sugar alcohols?

Here is an excerpt from a Nutrition Facts table providing information on the carbohydrate content

Carbohydrates	19 g
Sugars	3 g
Sorbitol	16 g

Practically speaking, despite the notable differences between them, one rule applies to nearly all sugar alcohols: Because only half of sugar alcohols is digested or absorbed, their carbohydrate content must be divided by two and subtracted from the total carbohydrate count.

- 16 g of sorbitol ÷ 2 = 8 g of carbohydrates not absorbed
- 19 g total carbohydrates – 8 g of unabsorbed sorbitol = 11 g of carbohydrates

Nevertheless, people on the basal-prandial regimen for variable-carbohydrate diets are not advised to include sugar alcohols in the carbohydrate count.

Because of their physiological properties, lactitol and polydextrose are not absorbed at all and their carbohydrate content should be subtracted in total from the food item's carbohydrate count.

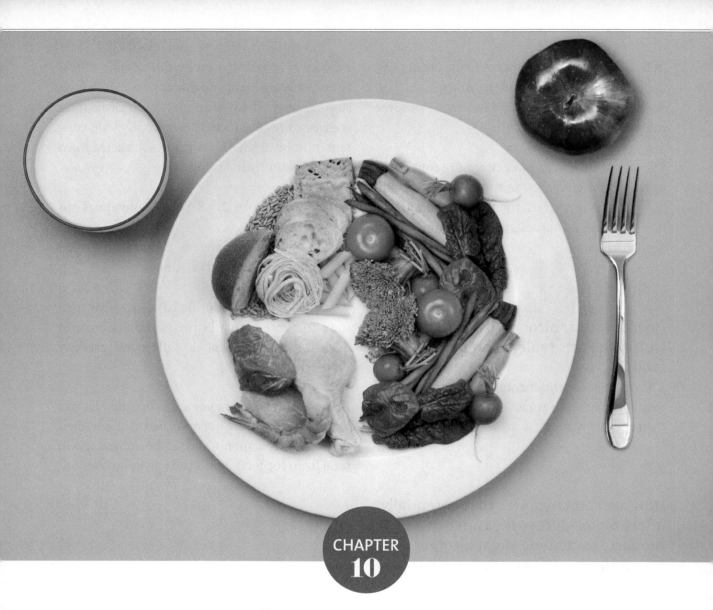

Planning
Meals

What are the benefits of meal-planning for people with diabetes?

Meal-planning can be of particular benefit to people with diabetes, helping them control their weight, blood glucose, blood pressure, and cholesterol levels.

How should meals be planned?

Having diabetes does not mean eating the same, boring food every day. By choosing an appropriate planning tool, people with diabetes can keep eating their favourite foods while introducing new items into their diets. Two meal planning tools based on the exchange system (*see chapter 7*) can help. They are:

- the meal plan;
- the plate method.

What is a meal plan?

A meal plan is a list of amounts of specific foods that correspond to your energy needs. It should also be compatible with your tastes, eating habits, schedule, medication, and any other illnesses associated with diabetes (high blood pressure, dyslipidemia and heart problems). A nutritionist can help you draw up your own personalized meal plan.

Nutrition plans indicate the amount of carbohydrates that should be in each meal and snack, as well as the number of servings of foods from the meat and alternatives group and the fats group your meals should contain.

It can be used as a model for daily meals, ensuring that you eat the same amount of carbohydrates from day to day and helping you control your blood glucose, while letting you vary your diet.

Here is an example of a meal plan for a meal:

SAMPLE MENU	
Dinner	
Starches	3 servings (45 g of carbohydrates)
Fruit	1 serving (15 g of carbohydrates)
Vegetables	2 servings
Milk	1 serving (15 g of carbohydrates)
Meat and alternatives	3 servings
Fats	1 serving

What is the plate method?

The plate method is easy to use. Even without a meal plan, the plate method can help you build a balanced meal containing foods from all groups.

Here are the five steps to creating a healthy plate:

Imagine your plate is subdivided into three sections.

1. Fill half of the plate with various vegetables such as spinach, carrots, eggplant, cauliflower, and tomatoes.

2. In one of the smaller sections, add starches such as whole-wheat bread, brown rice, pasta, potatoes, legumes, or corn.

3. In the other smaller section, add meat or a meat alternative such as skinned chicken, fish, seafood, lean beef, or tofu.

4. Add one serving of low-fat dairy such as milk or yogurt.

5. Finish it off with a serving of fruit.

Here is an illustration of a healthy plate:

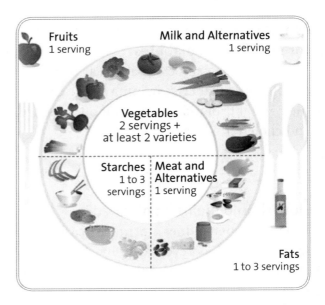

From *Meal Planning for People with Diabetes*, Quebec Ministère de la Santé et des Services sociaux.

A major benefit of this plan is that it helps reduce serving sizes of meat, meat alternatives, and starches, while encouraging vegetable consumption.

This meal contains between **45 g and 75 g of carbohydrates**.

Remember that you can use your hand as a useful tool to determine serving sizes. For example:

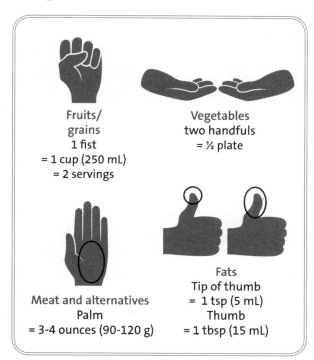

Fruits/ grains
1 fist
= 1 cup (250 mL)
= 2 servings

Vegetables
two handfuls
= ½ plate

Meat and alternatives
Palm
= 3-4 ounces (90-120 g)

Fats
Tip of thumb
= 1 tsp (5 mL)
Thumb
= 1 tbsp (15 mL)

How can I reduce a recipe's carbohydrate, fat, and sodium content?

Changing a few ingredients and the preparation method can improve the nutritional value of a recipe. For example, reduce the amount of some ingredients and substitute them with others with lower carbohydrate, fat, or sodium content.

Read the ingredients carefully to determine which ones can be changed to make a healthier dish.

To cut carbohydrate content:
- reduce the amount of sugar, honey, syrup, or dried fruit.
- use sugar substitutes like Splenda® (for cooking).
- use the same recipe but increase the number of servings.
- replace icing, fondant, or other rich garnishes with fruit coulis, Greek yogurt, or fresh fruit.

To cut fat content:
- skim the fat from the surface of cooled sauces and broths.
- replace some of the fats in a cake or muffin with fruit puree or yogurt.
- replace cream with unsweetened condensed milk.
- replace cream on fresh fruit with balsamic vinegar or a splash of port wine.

For cooking methods, see chapter 8.

To cut sodium:
- use fresh or dried herbs, spices, aromatics, or condiments such as garlic, ginger, or hot peppers.
- replace salt-based seasoning such as onion salt with a homemade salt substitute (*see recipe below*).
- taste before adding salt.
- choose low-sodium versions, if available (e.g., broth).
- choose fresh or frozen fruit or vegetables and homemade meals made with unprocessed foods instead of canned or pre-prepared food.

Homemade salt substitute

- 15 mL (1 tbsp) dry mustard
- 15 mL (1 tbsp) onion powder
- 15 mL (1 tbsp) garlic powder
- 15 mL (1 tbsp) paprika
- 3 mL (¾ tsp) ground black pepper
- 5 mL (1 tsp) ground basil
- 5 mL (1 tsp) ground thyme

A few practical tips

- Use homemade spice mixes or low-sodium commercial brands like Mrs. Dash® or McCormick® instead of salt substitutes, which are frequently high in potassium.
- When using herbs in a dish for the first time, add only a little and taste before adding any more.
- When cooking vegetables, add herbs at the beginning.
- It is recommended to consume less than 2300 mg of sodium per day.

For more information, see
www.sodium101.ca.

How can the carbohydrate value of one serving of a recipe be calculated for the purposes of the meal plan?

If the meal plan is based on 15 g servings of carbohydrates, you must determine how many servings a dish has. Take, for example, one prune muffin containing 28 g of carbohydrates:

$$28 \text{ g} \div 15 \text{ g} = 1.9 = 2 \text{ servings of 15 g each}$$

Know your meal plan well so you can identify the group your dishes belongs to.

In this example, the prune muffin can be counted as one 15 g serving of fruit and one 15 g serving of starch.

It also contains fats. Since foods in the starch or fruit groups are not sources of fat, this muffin also provides a fat serving that must be counted in the meal plan for the day.

In our example, one muffin equals one serving of fruit, one serving of starch, and one serving of fats. The meal needs to be completed with one serving of milk, two more servings of starch, three servings of meat or alternatives, and two servings of vegetables.

If the meal plan distributes a fixed amount of carbohydrates for each meal, the carbohydrate content of the muffins consumed must be counted, after which the carbohydrates required to reach the recommended amount should be added.

What if the number of servings and the nutritional value of a recipe are unknown? How can I figure out its carbohydrate content?

If you do not know the nutritional value of a recipe, it can be calculated from the list of ingredients, using a food composition table. For carbohydrate content, divide the total value of carbohydrates according to this table by the number of servings the recipe gives you.

You can also use a recipe analyzer such as ProFilAN. This tool is provided by the Dietitians of Canada (*see chapter 28 on "Resources" for the website*).

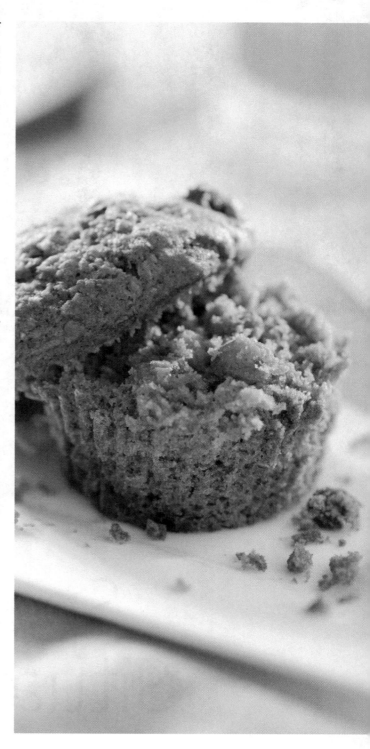

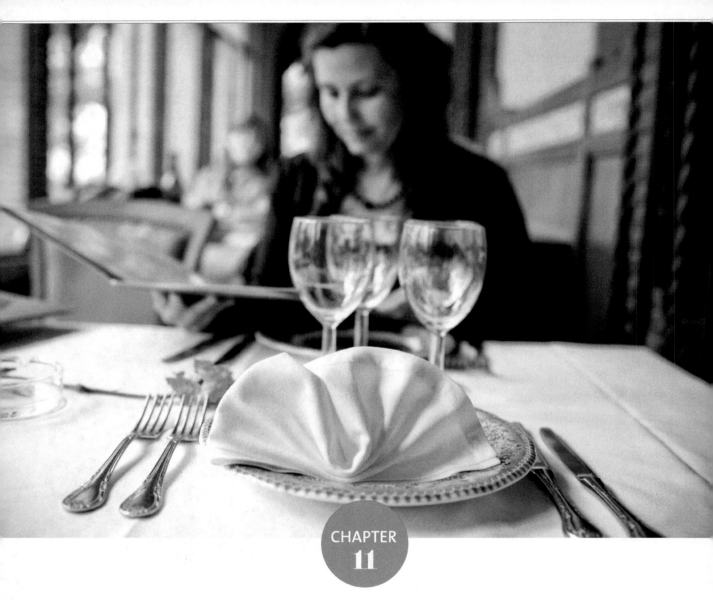

Special Situations

EATING OUT

Can people with diabetes go out to eat?

Yes. Occasional restaurant dining is one of life's pleasures, and diabetes should not be a reason to eliminate it. People with diabetes simply have to find ways to follow their nutrition plan while dining out.

Even if you eat out every day (e.g., lunch near the office), blood glucose levels can still be managed, so long as you make careful choices about what and how much you eat. When making these choices, it is important to remember that the fat content of restaurant food is on average 20% to 25% higher than foods you prepare at home, and that in many cases restaurants meals are not particularly balanced. Restaurant food is also generally higher in sodium (salt) and calories. Some restaurants display the nutritional value of their dishes in the menu or on their website.

How should people with diabetes choose a meal from a restaurant menu?

There are a number of different approaches to planning your meal in a restaurant.

- Know your nutrition plan.
- Find out about the ingredients or cooking method of the dishes that interest you.
- Choose all of your carbohydrates first, from the starter to the dessert, before ordering. Select a dish that is easy to assess just by looking at it (e.g., grilled meat) instead of something fried or a dish with sauce. This will make it easier to stick to your nutrition plan by having the proper amounts from each food group.
- Pay particular attention to serving size.
- Order food prepared with a minimum of fat, such as grilled or skewered meats or poached fish.
- Do not eat chicken skin, and avoid breaded or fried foods.
- Ask for sauces and salad dressing on the side whenever possible.
- Share your French fries, cake or pizza with your dining companion, or get a doggie bag.
- Order half-servings or items from the children's menu, if possible.
- Order two starters instead of a starter and a main course.

DELAYED MEALS

How are blood glucose levels affected if a meal is delayed?

A delayed meal can lead to hypoglycemia if the person with diabetes injects insulin or takes medications that stimulate the pancreas to produce more insulin (for example, glyburide, gliclazide, repaglinide).

One-hour delay: have a snack providing 5 g of carbohydrates at the scheduled mealtime and subtract this amount from the usual carbohydrate content of the meal.

Two- to three-hour delay: have the equivalent of one or two servings of starches (15 g to 30 g of carbohydrates) with a small amount of protein. Then subtract these servings from the eventual meal or, if the delayed meal is dinner, have the meal instead of the evening snack.

With the delayed meal, take oral antidiabetic medications to stimulate the pancreas to produce more insulin (e.g., glyburide, gliclazide, repaglinide) or insulin.

To visually estimate serving sizes for each food group in your nutrition plan, practice at home by measuring and weighing different foods and noticing how much room these foods take up in your plate. This can help you learn how to estimate servings with your hands (see chapter 10). To learn more, talk to your dietitian.

ALCOHOL

Can people with diabetes drink alcohol?

People with diabetes can drink alcohol if their diabetes is well controlled. Remember, however, that excessive alcohol consumption can affect blood glucose levels and can cause increases in:

- blood pressure;
- triglycerides;
- weight.

How does alcohol affect blood glucose?

There are two types of alcoholic drinks:

1 **Alcoholic drinks containing sugar:** These include beer, aperitif wines, and sweet wines. They can raise blood glucose.

2 **Alcoholic drinks that do not contain sugar:** These include dry wines and distilled alcohol such as gin, rye, rum, whisky, vodka, cognac, brandy, and so on. They do not raise blood glucose if they are consumed in small quantities.

For people with type 2 diabetes, drinking alcohol on an empty stomach can cause hypoglycemia, particularly for those who take insulin or medications to stimulate the pancreas to produce insulin (e.g., glyburide, gliclazide, repaglinide). For people with type 1 diabetes, moderate alcohol consumption with dinner or two to three hours after dinner can trigger delayed hypoglycemia the next morning or up to 24 hours later.

To avoid this risk:

- Have a snack before going to bed.
- Check blood glucose during the night, if recommended.

If I drink alcohol, what should I keep in mind?

- Alcohol has a **high calorie content**. Regular consumption can hamper weight loss or even cause weight gain because of the additional calories it provides.
- Alcohol is **not a part of any of the food groups in your nutrition plan**. Excessive drinking can be harmful to your health, especially if nutritious foods are left out of your regular meals.
- Excessive drinking can increase **triglycerides** (a type of blood lipid) and **blood pressure**.

What are the most important recommendations about alcohol?

1 Drink alcohol only if your diabetes is well controlled.

2 Drink alcohol with food, never on an empty stomach.

3 Drink in moderation:
- Women: 0 to 2 standard drinks per day (a maximum of 10 per week);
- Men: 0 to 3 standard drinks per day (a maximum of 15 per week).

4 Drink slowly.

5 Avoid drinking alcohol before, during or after physical activity.

One drink equals:
- 1½ oz (43 mL) of 40% (80 proof) spirits
- 5 oz (142 mL) of 12% wine
- 3 oz (86 mL) of 20% fortified wine
- 12 oz (341 mL) of 6% beer
- 2 x 5 oz (142 mL) of 6% cider

Remember:
- Just one drink can cause hypoglycemia.
- Just one drink is enough to make your breath smell like alcohol.
- Because the symptoms of hypoglycemia and drunkenness are very similar, people around you may confuse the two and delay appropriate treatment. Wear a bracelet or a pendant around your neck identifying you as having diabetes.

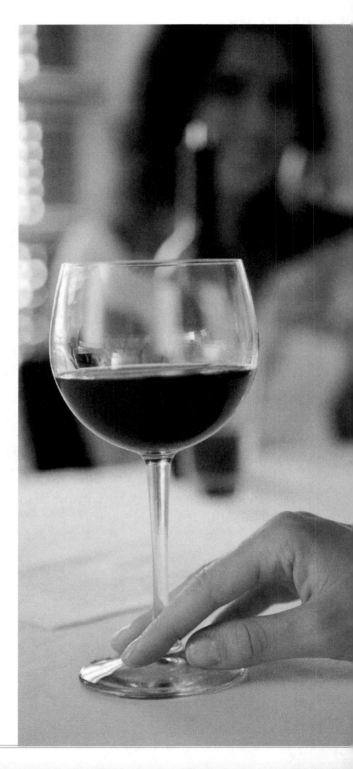

How many calories and carbohydrates do alcoholic drinks contain?

The following chart presents the calorie and carbohydrate contents of some alcoholic drinks.

Alcoholic drink	Quantity	Energy (calories)	Carbohydrates (grams)
Regular beer	341 mL (12 oz)	150	13
Light beer	341 mL (12 oz)	95	4
0.5% beer	341 mL (12 oz)	60 to 85	12 to 18
Low-carb beer	341 mL (12 oz)	90	2.5
Wine cooler	341 mL (12 oz)	170	22
Vodka Ice®	341 mL (12 oz)	260	50
Sweet sherry	56 mL (2 oz)	79	4
Sweet vermouth	56 mL (2 oz)	96	10
Scotch, rum, vodka, gin	43 mL (1½ oz)	98	0
Dry white wine	142 mL (5 oz)	106	1
Dry red wine	142 mL (5 oz)	106	2
Champagne	142 mL (5 oz)	120	2.5
Port	56 mL (2 oz)	91	7
Coffee liqueur	43 mL (1½ oz)	159	17
Cognac	43 mL (1½ oz)	112	0
Apple cider	142 mL (5 oz)	74 to 94	18 to 22

What are some alternatives to alcoholic drinks?

Alcoholic drinks can be replaced with:

- low-sodium carbonated water;
- diet soft drinks;
- tomato juice with lemon or Tabasco® sauce;
- iced water with lemon.

MINOR ILLNESSES

What effects do minor illnesses have on diabetes?

Minor illnesses such as a cold, the flu or gastroenteritis put stress on the body, destabilizing and increasing blood glucose in people with diabetes. This occurs for two reasons:

- An increase in the secretion of certain hormones causes glucose stored in the liver to enter the bloodstream.
- These same hormones increase insulin resistance and prevent glucose from entering the cells.

These two reactions can lead to hyperglycemia.

Be careful

In people with type 1 diabetes, ketoacidosis can resemble gastroenteritis (both cause nausea and vomiting). Be sure to check your blood glucose and ketone bodies regularly (*see chapter on hyperglycemia*).

What precautions should be taken in the case of a minor illness?

People with diabetes who have a cold or the flu but are not ill enough to warrant a visit to the doctor should follow these five guidelines:

1 Continue taking oral or injectable antidiabetic medications or insulin. Insulin needs can increase during an illness. Doctors can provide a sliding scale based on blood glucose readings to adjust insulin dosage for patients on insulin injection treatment. There are several methods to establish correction doses on sick days. It is therefore important to draw up a personalized action plan with your doctor so that you know what doses to take, when to take them, and in what circumstances. Corrective doses use the same insulin as that used for meals (rapid- or short-acting).

2 Check blood glucose every 4 hours or more often, if necessary.

3 Check for ketone bodies in urine or blood if blood glucose is higher than 14 mmol/L.

4 Drink a lot of water to prevent dehydration.

5 Eat the recommended amount of easily digested carbohydrates in your meals and snacks.

Should the same precautions be taken for gastroenteritis?

Gastroenteritis generally causes diarrhea and vomiting, sometimes leading to dehydration and a loss of electrolytes such as sodium and potassium because sufferers are unable to eat or drink.

Important!!!

See your doctor or go to the emergency room if any of the following situations occur:

- If you have type 1 diabetes, your blood glucose is higher than 20 mmol/L and your ketone bodies are moderate or high (see chapter 2), with or without vomiting. If you have type 2 diabetes, your blood glucose is higher than 30 mmol/L.
- You are vomiting continually and cannot retain liquids.
- You have a fever with a temperature higher than 38.5°C (101.3°F) for more than 48 hours.

A three-phase approach is recommended to avoid dehydration, soothe the intestine, and reduce diarrhea and vomiting:

Phase 1: Liquid nutrients for the first 24 hours

Consume only liquids. Drink water, broth or bouillon at any time and as much as you want.

Every hour, drink liquids containing about 15 g of carbohydrates. If you have trouble tolerating large amounts every hour, try drinking 15 mL or 1 tablespoon every 15 minutes instead.

Commercially available oral rehydrating solutions such as Gastrolyte® and Pedialyte® can be helpful. Or try a homemade preparation: mix 250 mL (1 cup) of orange juice, the same amount of water, and 2 mL (½ tsp) of salt. One cup (250 mL) provides 15 g of carbohydrates.

Gradually replace these drinks with juice, flavoured gelatine, regular non-caffeinated and flat soft drinks, and nutritional supplements (such as Glucerna®, Resource Diabetic® or Boost Diabetic®, for example).

Phase 2: Low-residue foods (gentle on the large intestine)

Gradually add solid foods, increasing consumption by portions of 15 g of carbohydrates, until you reach the recommended carbohydrate content in your nutrition plan. For example:

- Fruit group: 1 small raw apple (grated), ½ a ripe banana, 125 mL (½ cup) unsweetened orange juice, etc.;
- Starch group: 2 rusks, 7 soda crackers, 4 melba toasts, 1 slice of toast, 75 mL (⅓ cup) of plain pasta or rice, etc.;
- Vegetable group: carrots, beets, asparagus, string or wax beans, etc.;
- Meat group: lean meats such as chicken or turkey breast, fish cooked without fat, mild cheese, etc.

Phase 3: Eat normally

Gradually resume your normal diet according to your nutrition plan, but continue to limit your intake of certain items:

- foods that produce intestinal gas such as corn, legumes (chickpeas, red beans, etc.), cabbage, onions, garlic, and raw vegetables;
- foods that are irritants, including anything fried or spiced, as well as chocolate, coffee, and cola.

TRIPS

How should a person with diabetes plan a trip?

When preparing for a trip, people with diabetes should take the following precautions:

- Make sure your diabetes is **well controlled**.
- Get a **doctor's letter** stating that you have diabetes and describing your treatment, particularly if you require insulin injections.
- Carry **identification** or a bracelet indicating that you have diabetes.
- Find out what coverage is provided by **insurance companies** for pre-existing diseases incurring medical expenses abroad. Also find out whether your travel insurance covers the cost of returning home in the event of a medical emergency.
- Find out about the **habits and customs** of the country you are visiting.
- **Inform the airline, railroad company, or bus line** that you have diabetes to find out what time meals are served and order a diabetic meal, if applicable.
- Find out about vaccines or any other treatments you need before you leave (e.g., malaria prevention) from a **travel clinic** or your doctor.
- Prepare a **travel health kit** with treatments for diarrhea, vomiting, and travel sickness. Include antibiotics if your doctor advises.
- Bring at least two pairs of **comfortable shoes**.
- **Do not travel alone.**

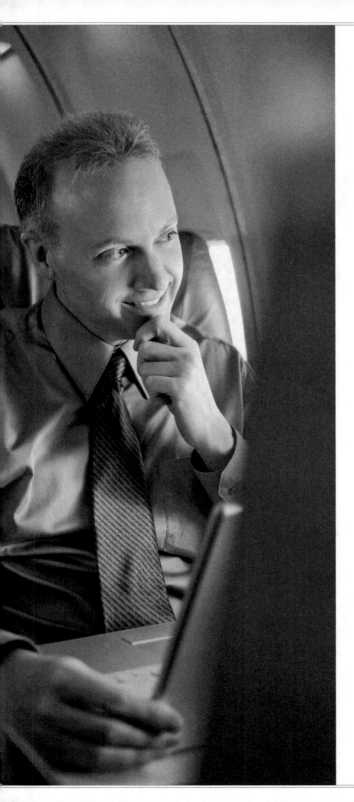

What precautions be taken when travelling with material and medication for treating diabetes?

Keep everything you need to treat your diabetes in a carry-on bag, not in your checked or stored luggage. Be sure that you have on hand:

- all of your medications with the label from the pharmacy to identify them.
- twice the normal amount of insulin you will need, in case vials break or you cannot find your insulin abroad. Be careful: in some countries, insulin is packaged and sold in a different concentration (40 units/ mL). When injecting, make sure the syringe corresponds to the concentration of insulin used.
- an insulating case to protect your insulin.
- extra syringes, even if you use a pen device.
- a self-monitoring kit (meter, test strips, etc.).
- emergency food provisions in case of hypoglycemia or a delayed meal (e.g., dried or fresh fruit, juice, nuts, packets of peanut butter, cheese and crackers) or glucose tablets.

Is there any special advice for travellers with diabetes?

When travelling, do the following:

- Follow your regular meal and snack schedule as closely as possible.
- Because your habits or routine could change, continue to check your blood glucose levels regularly to make sure your diabetes is still under control.
- Always carry food provisions in case of hypoglycemia or a delayed meal (for example, dried or fresh fruits, juice, nuts, packets of peanut butter, cheese and crackers, or glucose tablets).
- Check your feet daily for cuts or contusions, and avoid walking barefoot.

How should people on the split-mixed insulin regimen adapt their insulin doses for time differences of more than three hours?

The split-mixed insulin regimen is a combination of intermediate-acting (Humulin® N or Novolin® ge NPH) and rapid-acting (Apidra®, Humalog® or NovoRapid ®) or short-acting insulin (Humulin® R or Novolin® ge Toronto), injected before the morning and evening meals.

For example, the time difference between Montreal and Paris is six hours. Suppose you normally take the following insulin doses:

- Novolin® ge NPH 16 units and NovoRapid® (NR) 8 units before breakfast;
- Novolin® ge NPH 6 units and NovoRapid® (NR) 6 units before dinner.

Travelling from:

Montreal to Paris. The departure day will be six hours shorter, so **reduce your NPH dose by 50% before dinner. Eat only half of your dinner before leaving and the other half during the flight.** Take 50% of your NR dose before dinner in Montreal and **50% before the evening in-flight meal**.

Meal	Blood glucose	Insulin	Meal
Montreal: breakfast	yes	NPH 16 units NR 8 units	normal
Montreal: lunch	yes	----	normal
Montreal: dinner	yes	NPH 3 units NR 3 units	50%
In flight: evening meal	yes	NR 3 units	50%
In flight: breakfast	yes	NPH 16 units NR 8 units	normal

Travelling from:

Paris to Montreal. The return day will be six hours longer, so have your **in-flight dinner** with the regular amount of NR insulin. Also **have an additional evening meal** containing 50% of a regular dinner's carbohydrates, **preceded by a dose of NR equal to 50% of your usual pre-dinner dose.** The NPH dose should be delayed until the second evening meal.

Meal	Blood glucose	Insulin	Meal
Paris: breakfast	yes	NPH 16 units NR 8 units	normal
Paris: lunch	yes	----	normal
In flight: dinner	yes	NR 6 units	normal
Montreal: evening meal	yes	NPH 6 units NR 3 units	50 %

How should people on the basal-prandial insulin regimen with fixed carbohydrates adapt their insulin doses for time differences of more than three hours?

The basal-prandial regimen with a fixed-carbohydrate diet consists of one injection of rapid-acting (Apidra®, Humalog® or NovoRapid®) or short-acting (Humulin® R or Novolin® ge Toronto) insulin before each meal and one injection of intermediate-acting (Humulin® N or Novolin® ge NPH) or long-acting (Levemir® or Lantus®) insulin at bedtime.

For example, the time difference between Montreal and Paris is six hours. Suppose you normally take the following insulin doses:
- NovoRapid® (NR) 8 units before breakfast;
- NovoRapid® (NR) 8 units before lunch;
- NovoRapid® (NR) 8 units before dinner;
- Novolin® ge NPH 8 units before bedtime.

Because of the extended action time of the long-acting insulin (Levemir® or Lantus®), there is no need to change the dose.

Travelling from:

Montreal to Paris. The departure day will be six hours shorter, so **move up your NPH insulin dose to before dinner and take only 50% of it.** Have **half of your dinner carbohydrates before leaving and the other half during the in-flight evening meal.** Also take **50% of your NR dose before dinner in Montreal and 50% before the in-flight evening meal.**

Note that because the day is six hours shorter, the Lantus® or Levemir® dose should be taken earlier, before leaving.

Travelling from:

Paris to Montreal. The return day will be six hours longer, so **have your in-flight dinner** with the regular amount of NR insulin. You should also **eat an additional evening meal** containing 50% of your usual dinner carbohydrates, **preceded by 50% of your usual pre-dinner NR dose.**

In addition, delay the NPH dose until bedtime. Lantus® or Levemir® should be taken at bedtime as usual.

Meal	Blood glucose	Insulin	Meal
Montreal: breakfast	Yes	NR 8 units	normal
Montreal: lunch	Yes	NR 8 units	normal
Montreal: dinner	yes	NPH 4 units NR 4 units	50%
In flight: evening meal	yes	NR 4 units	50%
In flight: breakfast	yes	NR 8 units	normal

Meal	Blood glucose	Insulin	Meal
Paris: breakfast	Yes	NR 8 units	normal
Paris: lunch	Yes	NR 8 units	normal
In flight: dinner	Yes	NR 8 units	normal
Montreal: evening meal	Yes	NR 4 units	50%
Montreal: bedtime snack	Yes	NPH 8 units	snack

6

How should people on the basal-prandial insulin regimen with variable carbohydrates adapt their insulin doses for time differences of more than three hours?

The basal-prandial insulin regimen with variable carbohydrate intake consists of one injection of rapid-acting (Apidra®, Humalog® or NovoRapid®) or short-acting (Humulin® R or Novolin® ge Toronto) insulin before each meal and one injection of intermediate-acting (Humulin® N or Novolin® ge NPH) or long-acting (Levemir® or Lantus®) insulin at bedtime.

For example, the time difference between Montreal and Paris is six hours. Suppose you normally take the following insulin doses:
- Humalog® (Hg) 1.2 units/10 g of carbohydrates before breakfast;
- Humalog® (Hg) 1.0 unit/10 g of carbohydrates before lunch;
- Humalog® (Hg) 1.0 unit/10 g of carbohydrates before the evening meal;
- Lantus® 12 units at bedtime.

Because long-acting insulin (Lantus®) has an extended action time, it is not necessary to change the dose.

Travelling from:

Montreal to Paris. The departure day will be six hours shorter, so the **Lantus® dose should be taken earlier, before you leave.** Although people on the basal-prandial insulin regimen with variable carbohydrate intake can wait to eat dinner on the plane, **a light meal before departure is recommended**, along with **Hg insulin** according to the amount of carbohydrates consumed. An in-flight evening meal is also possible, again with Hg insulin according to the amount of carbohydrates consumed, at the same dose as taken for dinner. **The next morning, the usual Hg insulin dose should be taken before the in-flight breakfast.**

Meal	Blood glucose	Insulin	Meal
Montreal: breakfast	yes	Hg 1.2 unit/ 10 g of carbohydrates	normal
Montreal: lunch	yes	Hg 1.0 unit/ 10 g of carbohydrates	normal
Montreal: dinner	yes	Lantus 12 units; Hg 1.0 unit/ 10 g of carbohydrates	50%
In flight: evening meal	yes	Hg 1.0 unit/10 g of carbohydrates	normal or 50%
In flight: breakfast	yes	Hg 1.2 unit/10 g of carbohydrates	normal

Travelling from:

Paris to Montreal. The return day will be six hours longer, so have **your in-flight dinner with the usual dose of Hg insulin, and have an additional evening meal**, along with the usual pre-dinner dose of Hg. **Take Lantus® at bedtime as usual.**

Meal	Blood glucose	Insulin	Meal
Paris: breakfast	yes	Hg 1.2 unit/ 10 g of carbohydrates	normal
Paris: lunch	yes	Hg 1.0 unit/ 10 g of carbohydrates	normal
In flight: dinner	yes	Hg 1.0 unit/ 10 g of carbohydrates	normal
Montreal: evening meal	yes	Hg 1.0 unit/ 10 g of carbohydrates	normal or 50%
Montreal: bedtime snack	yes	Lantus 12 units	snack

How should people on the premixed insulin regimen adapt their insulin doses for time differences of more than three hours?

The premixed insulin regimen consists of one injection of a mix of rapid-acting or short-acting insulin and intermediate-acting insulin (Humulin® 30/70, Novolin® ge 30/70, 50/50, 40/60, Humalog® Mix 25, etc.) before breakfast and dinner.

For example, the time difference between Montreal and Paris is six hours. Suppose you normally take the following doses of Humulin® 30/70:

- 20 units before breakfast;
- 10 units before dinner.

Travelling from:

Montreal to Paris. The departure day will be six hours shorter, so **have half of your dinner carbohydrates before leaving and the other half during the flight. Also take half of your insulin dose at dinner before you leave and the other half before the in-flight evening meal.**

Travelling from:

Paris to Montreal. The return day will be six hours longer, so **have an additional evening meal** (50% of the usual carbohydrate content) **preceded by a dose of insulin equivalent to 50% of the usual pre-dinner dose.**

Meal	Blood glucose	Insulin	Meal
Montreal: breakfast	yes	H 30/70 20 units	normal
Montreal: lunch	yes	---	normal
Montreal: dinner	yes	H 30/70 5 units	50%
In flight: evening meal	yes	H 30/70 5 units	50%
In flight: breakfast	yes	H 30/70 20 units	normal

Meal	Blood glucose	Insulin	Meal
Paris: breakfast	yes	H 30/70 20 units	normal
Paris: lunch	yes	----	normal
In flight: dinner	yes	H 30/70 10 units	normal
Montreal: evening meal	yes	H 30/70 5 units	50%
Montreal: bedtime snack	yes	----	snack

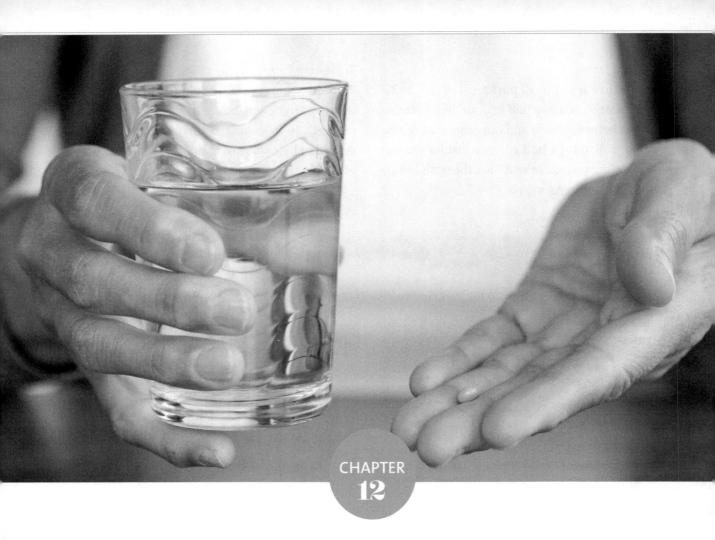

Antidiabetic Drugs other than Insulin

What are antidiabetic drugs?

Antidiabetic drugs are medications that lower blood glucose levels. Some antidiabetic drugs are taken orally, while others are injected subcutaneously.

When should antidiabetic drugs be used to treat diabetes?

Antidiabetic drugs are used to treat type 2 diabetes if diet, exercise, and weight loss programs are not sufficient to normalize blood glucose levels. They can be taken alone or in combination.

WARNING! Antidiabetic drugs are complementary treatments. They do not replace diet, exercise and weight loss programs.

What antidiabetic drugs are available in Canada?

There are approximately twenty antidiabetic drugs on the market in Canada. They are grouped into different classes:

CLASS	DRUG (Name generic/brand)
oral antidiabetic drugs	
Sulfonylureas*	• Chlorpropamide (e.g., Apo®- Chlorpropamide) • Gliclazide (e.g., Diamicron®) • Glimepiride (e.g., Amaryl®) • Glyburide (Diaßeta®, Euglucon®) • Tolbutamide (e.g., Apo®-Tolbutamide)
Meglitinides*	• Nateglinide (Starlix®) • Repaglinide (e.g., GlucoNorm®)
Biguanides	• Metformin (e.g., Glucophage®)
Thiazolidinediones	• Pioglitazone (Actos®) • Rosiglitazone (Avandia®)
Alpha-glucosidase inhibitors	• Acarbose (Glucobay®)
Dipeptidyl peptidase-4 (DPP-4) inhibitors**	• Linagliptin (Trajenta ®) • Saxagliptin (Onglyza®) • Sitagliptin (Januvia®)
Injectable antidiabetic drugs	
GLP-1 agonists**	• Exenatide (Byetta®) • Liraglutide (Victoza®)

*Insulin secretagogues
** Incretin agents. GLP-1 (glucagon-like peptide-1)

What are the characteristics of sulfonylureas such as glyburide (Diaßeta®), glicazide (Diamicron®), and glimepiride (Amaryl®)?

- **Mechanism of action:** Sulfonylureas stimulate the pancreas to produce more insulin (they are insulin secretagogues). They are therefore ineffective if the insulin-producing cells of the pancreas no longer function.

- **Adverse effects:** Hypoglycemia is the adverse effect most commonly attributed to sulfonylureas. It can occur at any time of day or night; dosage should therefore be adjusted accordingly. To minimize the risk of hypoglycemia, meals and snacks should be eaten on a regular schedule as set out in the meal plan. Sulfonylureas should not be taken at bedtime.

- **When to take them:** Sulfonylureas should be taken before meals, but never more than 30 minutes beforehand. Sulfonylureas that are taken once a day – for example, modified release gliclazide (Diamicron® MR) and glimepiride (Amaryl®) – should be taken with breakfast.

What are the characteristics of the meglitinides nateglinide (Starlix®) and repaglinide (GlucoNorm®)?

- **Mechanism of action:** Like sulfonylureas, nateglinide and repaglinide stimulate the pancreas to produce more insulin (they are insulin secretagogues). They are therefore ineffective if the insulin-producing cells of the pancreas no longer function. They are faster and shorter acting than sulfonylureas.

- **Adverse effects:** Hypoglycemia is the adverse effect most commonly attributed to nateglinide and repaglinide. Dosage should be adjusted accordingly. To minimize the risk of hypoglycemia, meals and snacks should be eaten on a regular schedule as set out in the meal plan. Nateglinide and repaglinide should not be taken at bedtime.

- **When to take them:** They should be taken as close as possible to the beginning of a meal (0 to 15 minutes), but never more than 30 minutes beforehand.

What are the characteristics of biguanides such as metformin (Glucophage®)?

- **Mechanism of action:** The primary action of metformin is to reduce the production of glucose by the liver. It also lowers insulin resistance or, in other words, improve insulin action.
- **Adverse effects:** Intestinal problems, especially diarrhea, are the side effects most commonly attributed to metformin. These adverse side effects can be reduced by beginning treatment slowly and gradually increasing your doses. Some patients also note a slight metallic aftertaste. When taken on its own, metformin is very rarely associated with hypoglycemia.
- **When to take it:** Take metformin at mealtime in order to minimize adverse intestinal effects.

What are the characteristics of thiazolidinediones e.g., pioglitazone (Actos®) and rosiglitazone (Avandia®)?

- **Mechanism of action:** Pioglitazone and rosiglitazone lower insulin resistance or in other words, increase the effectiveness of insulin. This results in an increase in the use of glucose by muscle tissue in particular and by adipose (fatty) tissue.
- **Adverse effects:** Edema (swelling due to water retention) and weight gain are possible adverse effects. People with cardiovascular disease should use these drugs with caution or avoid them altogether. Rosiglitazone has been associated with an increased risk of non-fatal myocardial infarction (heart attack), and pioglitazone may be associated with an increased risk of bladder cancer. Both increase the risk of bone fracture in women. As a result, the use of thiazolidinediones is currently quite limited. When taken on their own, pioglitazone and rosiglitazone are generally not associated with hypoglycemia.
- **When to take them:** These drugs should always be taken at the same time of day, usually in the morning. They do not have to be taken with meals.

What are the characteristics of alpha-glucosidases inhibitors such as acarbose (Glucobay®)?

- **Mechanism of action:** Acarbose slows the absorption of carbohydrates ingested at meals thus controlling the rising of blood glucose levels after meals.
- **Adverse effects:** The adverse effects most commonly attributed to acarbose are intestinal problems, particularly bloating and flatulence (gas). When taken on its own, acarbose is not associated with hypoglycemia.
- **When to take it:** To ensure effectiveness, acarbose should be taken with the first mouthful of a meal.

What are the characteristics of DPP-4 inhibitors such as linagliptin (Trajenta®), saxagliptin (Onglyza®), and sitagliptin (Januvia®)?

- **Mechanism of action:** DPP-4 inhibitors intensify the effect of certain intestinal hormones (such as GLP-1) involved in the control of blood sugar. It causes an increase in insulin secretion and a decrease in the secretion of glucagon (a hyperglycemic hormone), but only if blood sugar is high.
- **Adverse effects:** DDP-4 inhibitors are generally well tolerated. When taken alone, a DPP-4 inhibitor is very rarely associated with hypoglycemia.
- **When to take it:** This drug should always be taken at the same time of day, usually in the morning. It is not necessary to take it with food.

What are the characteristics of GLP-1 agonists such as exenatie (Byetta®) and liraglutide (Victoza®)?

- **Mechanism of action:** Exenatide and liraglutide mimic the effect of certain intestinal hormones known as incretins (such as GLP-1) involved in the control of blood glucose. They cause an increase in the secretion of insulin and a decrease in the secretion of glucagon (a hyperglycemic hormone), but only if blood glucose is high. They also decrease the speed of the emptying of the stomach and reduce appetite. They can be associated with weight loss. These drugs are injected subcutaneously.
- **Adverse effects:** Nausea, diarrhea, vomiting and headache are the main undesirable side effects of GLP-1 agonists. When taken alone, this class of agent is very rarely associated with hypoglycemia.
- **When to take it:** Exenatide should be taken within the hour before breakfast and supper. Liraglutide is taken once daily at the same time every day.
- **Other considerations:** GLP-1 agonists are injected subcutaneously with a pre-filled pen injector with a screw-on needle (like insulin). Unused pen injectors should be stored in the refrigerator and will remain stable until the date of expiry. Pen injectors in use should be stored at room temperature (maximum 25° for Byetta® and 30°C for Victoza®) and can be kept for 30 days.

What should be done if a dose is missed?

- If you notice the omission quickly, take the dose immediately. If not, skip the missed dose and wait for the next one scheduled.
- **Never double the dose.**
- It is not a good idea to take sulfonylureas, nateglinide or repaglinide at bedtime, as they can cause a risk of nocturnal hypoglycemia.
- Acarbose is effective only if it is taken with a meal. If forgotten at mealtime, there is no point in taking it afterwards.
- Exenatide (Byetta®) must be taken within the hour before breakfast and supper. It must not be taken after meals. If the morning dose is forgotten, it can be taken before lunch as long as there are six hours between it and the before-supper dose.

Why is it often necessary to take several antidiabetic drugs at the same time?

Any given class of antidiabetic drugs has its own particular mechanism of action. Secretagogues, for example, stimulate the release of insulin via the pancreas, while biguanides decrease the production of glucose by the liver. In many cases, combining agents with different mechanisms of action can increase the effectiveness of treatment. Some drugs are available in pills combining two drugs.

How do I choose the antidiabetic drug that is best for me?

Follow recommendations for the treatment of diabetes based on current scientific data. The choice of drug for a specific individual should also take into account factors including blood sugar, glycated hemoglobin, age, how long the person has had diabetes, and other health problems.

Do oral antidiabetic drugs interact with other medications?

All drugs can potentially interact with other agents. The responsibility for anticipating and preventing such interactions falls on pharmacists and doctors, but the patient also has a role to play.

People taking medication should keep an up-to-date list of their prescriptions, ideally one provided by their pharmacist. They are strongly advised to bring their medication containers with them when seeing the doctor, who will use them to guide any decisions about treatment. It is also a good idea for people with diabetes to use the same pharmacist at all times; in such a case, the pharmacist will be better able to detect potential problems (duplicate prescriptions, adverse effects, or interactions, for example) and advise appropriately.

Are oral antidiabetic drugs long-term treatments?

At this point, diabetes is a disease that can be controlled but not cured. Generally speaking, therefore, oral antidiabetic drugs are long-term treatments. Your doctor will regularly adjust your treatment, either increasing or decreasing dosages. The goal of the treatment is to normalize blood glucose levels without causing adverse effects such as hypoglycemia.

MECHANISM OF ACTION OF ORAL ANTIDIABETIC DRUGS

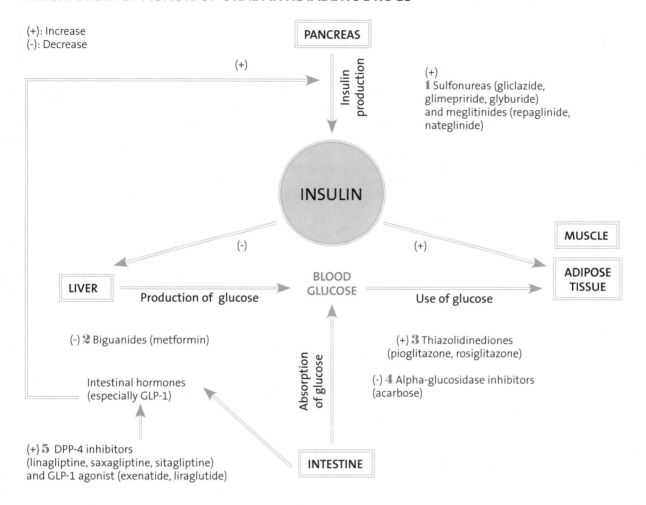

(+): Increase
(-): Decrease

PANCREAS

Insulin production

(+)

(+)
1 Sulfonureas (gliclazide, glimepriride, glyburide) and meglitinides (repaglinide, nateglinide)

INSULIN

MUSCLE

ADIPOSE TISSUE

(-)

(+)

LIVER

Production of glucose

BLOOD GLUCOSE

Use of glucose

(-) **2** Biguanides (metformin)

(+) **3** Thiazolidinediones (pioglitazone, rosiglitazone)

(-) **4** Alpha-glucosidase inhibitors (acarbose)

Absorption of glucose

Intestinal hormones (especially GLP-1)

(+) **5** DPP-4 inhibitors (linagliptine, saxagliptine, sitagliptine) and GLP-1 agonist (exenatide, liraglutide)

INTESTINE

1 Sulfonylureas and meglitinides stimulate the pancreas to produce more insulin (insulin secretagogues).

2 Biguanides reduce the production of glucose by the liver.

3 Thiazolidinediones increase insulin action, which increases the use of glucose, especially by muscle tissue but also by adispose (fatty) tissue.

4 Alpha-glucosidase inhibitors delay the absorption of dietary carbohyrates.

5 DPP-4 inhibitors and GLP-1 agonists intensify the action of certain intestinal hormones such as GLP-1 that favour insulin secretion by the pancreas when blood glucose is high

N.B. See the table on the different antidiabetic medications for further information.

ORAL ANTIDIABETIC DRUGS

Drug	Glyburide	Gliclazide	Gliclazide modified release	Glimepiride	Repaglinide	Nateglinide
Class	Sulfonylurea (insulin secretagogue)	Sulfonylurea (insulin secretagogue)	Sulfonylurea (insulin secretagogue)	Sulfonylurea (insulin secretagogue)	Meglitinide (insulin secretagogue)	Meglitinide (insulin secretagogue)
Brand name (non-exhaustive list)	Diaßeta Euglucon Apo-Glyburide Mylan-Glybe Teva-Glyburide	Diamicron Ava-Gliclazide Novo-Gliclazide pms-Gliclazide	Diamicron MR Gliclazide MR	Amaryl Apo-Glimepiride Ratio-Glimepiride	GlucoNorm CO-Repaglinide pms-Repaglinide	Starlix
Format marketed	2.5 mg and 5 mg tablets (divisible into two)	80 mg tables (divisible into four)	30 mg and 60 mg tablets (30 mg indivisible; 60 mg divisible)	1 mg, 2 mg and 4 mg tablets (divisible into two)	0.5 mg, 1 mg and 2 mg (indivisible)	60 mg and 120 mg tablets (indivisible)
Daily dosage	1.25 mg to 20 mg	40 mg to 320 mg	30 mg to 120 mg	1 mg to 8 mg	1 mg to 16 mg	180 mg to 360 mg
Number of daily doses	1 to 3	1 to 3	1	1	2 to 4 (depending on the number of meals)	3
When to take it	0 to 30 min before meals	0 to 30 min before meals	At breakfast	At breakfast	0 to 15 min before meals	0 to 15 min before meals
Most common adverse effects	Hypoglycemia	Hypoglycemia	Hypoglycemia	Hypoglycemia	Hypoglycemia	Hypoglycemia
Risk of hypoglycemia	Yes	Yes	Yes	Yes	Yes	Yes

Acarbose	Metformin	Slow-release metformin	Pioglitazone	Rosiglitazone	Rosiglitazone and metformin
Alpha-glucosidase inhibitor	Biguanide	Biguanide	Thiazolidinedione	Thiazolidinedione	Thiazolidinedione and biguanide
Glucobay	Glucophage Apo-Metformin Jamp-Metformin Novo-Metformin Riva-Metformin	Glumetza	Actos Apo-pioglitazone Mint-pioglitazone Ran-pioglitazone	Avandia	Avandamet
50 mg and 100 mg tablets (divisible into two)	500 mg tablets (divisible into two) and 850 mg (indivisible)	500 mg tablets	15 mg, 30 mg and 45 mg tablets (indivisible)	2 mg, 4 mg and 8 mg tablets (indivisible)	2 mg/500 mg 4 mg/500 mg 2 mg/1000 mg 4 mg/1000 mg tablets (rosiglitazone/metformin) (indivisible)
50 mg to 300 mg	250 mg to 2500 mg	500 mg to 2000 mg	15 mg to 45 mg	4 mg to 8 mg	2 mg/1000 mg to 8 mg/2000 mg
1 to 3	1 to 4	1	1	1 to 2	2
With the first bite of a meal	At meals	At supper	With or without food	With or without food	At meals
Bloating, flatulence, diarrhea	Diarrhea / metallic taste	Diarrhea	Oedema / weight gain	Oedema / weight gain	Oedema / weight gain / diarrhea / metallic taste
No	No	No	No	No	No

Drug	Linagliptin	Saxagliptin	Sitagliptin	Linagliptin and metformin	Saxagliptin and metformin
Class	DPP-4 inhibitor	DPP-4 inhibitor	DPP-4 inhibitor	DPP-4 inhibitor and biguanide	DPP-4 inhibitor and biguanide
Brand name (non-exhaustive list)	Trajenta	Onglyza	Januvia	Jentadueto	Komboglyze
Format marketed	5 mg tablet (indivisble)	2.5 mg and 5 mg tablets (indivisible)	25 mg, 50 mg and 100 mg tablets (indivisible)	2.5 mg/500 mg 2.5 mg/850 mg 2.5 mg/1000 mg tablets	2.5 mg/500 mg 2.5 mg/850 mg 2.5 mg/1000 mg tablets
Daily dosage	5 mg	2.5 mg to 5 mg	25 mg to 100 mg	5 mg/1000mg 5 mg/2000mg	5 mg/1000 mg 5 mg/2000 mg
Number of daily doses	1	1	1	2	2
When to take it	With or without meal, at the same time daily	With or without meal, at the same time daily	With or without meal, at the same time daily	With meals	With meals
Most common adverse effects	Well tolerated	Well tolerated	Well tolerated	Diarrhea / metallic taste	Diarrhea / metallic taste
Risk of hypoglycemia	No	No	No	No	No

INJECTABLE ANTIDIABETIC DRUGS

Sitagliptin and metformin	Exenatide	Liraglutide
DPP-4 inhibitor and biguanide	GLP-1 agonist	GLP-1 agonist
Janumet	Byetta	Victoza
50 mg/500 mg 50 mg/850 mg 50 mg/1000 mg tablets	250 mcg/mL pen device: 5 mcg/dose (1.2 mL) and 10 mcg/dose (2.4 mL)	6 mg /mL (3 mL) pen device
100 mg/1000 mg 100 mg/2000 mg	10 mcg to 20 mcg	0.6 mg, 1.2 mg and 1.8 mg
2	2	1
With meals	Within the hour before breakfast and supper	At the same time daily
Diarrhea / metallic taste	Nausea, diarrhea, vomiting, headache	Nausea, diarrhea, vomiting, headache
No	No	No

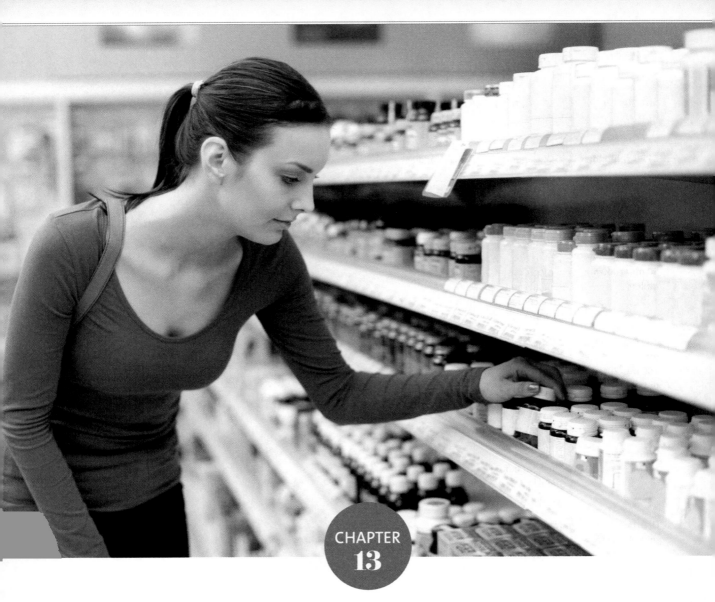

Over-the-Counter Drugs

What are over-the-counter drugs?

Over-the-counter drugs include all medications sold without prescription. Some can be obtained only after consulting a pharmacist, although most can be purchased on the spot.

When and how should over-the-counter drugs be used?

Over-the-counter drugs allow people to self-medicate for **mild health problems**. They should only be used for **short periods of time** to ensure that they are not masking the symptoms of a more serious condition. All directions and warnings printed on the packaging should be followed closely.

Are over-the-counter drugs free of side effects?

No drug is completely free of side effects. In some cases, over-the-counter drugs can cause adverse effects. Some drugs should be avoided or used with caution by people with certain illnesses. There is also a risk of interactions between over-the-counter and prescription drugs.

How can I be sure that the over-the-counter drugs I choose are safe?

It is strongly recommended that you speak with your pharmacist before selecting an over-the-counter drug. Your pharmacist can recommend the most suitable product, taking into account your symptoms, health problems, and any other drugs you are taking, possibly even suggesting non-pharmacological alternatives. The pharmacist will recommend that you see your doctor if he or she believes that your condition requires it. Always have your prescriptions filled by the same pharmacist; this will ensure that your file is always up-to-date and that the pharmacist has all the information necessary to properly advise you.

Which over-the-counter drugs should be avoided or used with caution by people with diabetes?

The following drugs should be used with caution:

- **oral decongestants** (for the treatment of nasal congestion);
- medications containing **sugar**;
- **keratolytic** preparations (for the treatment of corns, calluses and warts);
- high doses of **acetylsalicylic acid**/ASA (e.g., Aspirin®).

Why should oral decongestants be used with caution?

Oral decongestants (e.g., Sudafed®) are medications in syrup, tablet or powder form that reduce nasal congestion. Most oral decongestants contain what is known as a "sympathomimetic" ingredient (e.g., pseudoephedrine) that can have a **hyperglycemic** effect, especially if recommended doses are exceeded. These types of products are frequently overused. Cold medications often contain a mixture of ingredients (to relieve coughs, fight fever, etc.), including a sympathomimetic decongestant. It is not uncommon for people to take two different products when treating a cold or the flu, thereby unintentionally doubling the dosage of the decongestant.

This type of oral decongestant is also not recommended for people with vascular problems, high blood pressure, hyperthyroidism or heart diseases such as angina.

Recommended alternative treatments include drinking plenty of water, keeping the room humidified and using a saline nasal vaporizer. If the condition persists, a nasal decongestant vaporizer may be used, but for no longer than 72 hours (to avoid rebound congestion).

Why should drugs containing sugar be used cautiously?

People with diabetes need to know which drugs contain sugar so that they do not unintentionally hamper their control of their blood glucose levels. Sugar is found not only in syrups, but also in powders, chewable tablets, and lozenges, among other things. People with diabetes should avoid any medication containing more than **20 calories** (5 g of carbohydrates) **per dose or providing more than 80 calories** (20 g of carbohydrates) **per day**. If these amounts are exceeded, they should be included in the overall carbohydrate tally of the meal plan. If the sugar content of a product is not printed on the packaging, the pharmacist can provide this information.

A number of "sucrose-free" or "sugar-free" preparations are also available. They usually contain sugar substitutes and can be used by people with diabetes at the recommended dose, as long as the active ingredient is not contraindicated for another reason.

Why should keratolytic preparations (for the treatment of corns, calluses and warts) be used with caution?

Adhesive plasters, pads, ointments or gels containing products such as salicylic or tannic acid are often used to treat corns, calluses and warts. These acids are highly irritating. See a doctor, a podiatrist or a nurse specializing in foot care before using these products.

Why should high doses of acetylsalicylic acid be used with caution?

Acetylsalicylic acid, also known as ASA (e.g., Aspirin®, Anacin®, Entrophen®, etc.) can cause **hypoglycemia** if taken daily in doses exceeding 3000 mg – the equivalent of more than 9 tablets of 325 mg per day or more than 6 tablets of 500 mg per day.

Acetaminophen (e.g., Tylenol®, Atasol®, etc.) does not contain acetylsalicylic acid and is a safe alternative to relieve fever and pain.

When shopping at the pharmacy, is there a simple way to determine which over-the-counter drugs should be used with caution or avoided?

In Quebec, the Ordre des pharmaciens du Québec has developed a program called the "Code médicament" ("Drug Caution Code"). It consists of six letters, each letter corresponding to a specific warning. These code letters usually appear on the price sticker or the shelf where the medication is placed.

Code letter "E" specifically concerns people with diabetes. Products bearing an "E" are **not recommended**. There are three types:
1) oral decongestants;
2) drugs with a sugar content in the recommended dose equalling 20 calories or more **per dose** or 80 calories or more **per day**;
3) keratolytic preparations (for the treatment of corns, calluses and warts).

In Quebec, a personalized card from your pharmacist will indicate the code letters that apply to you.

If you are not in Quebec, ask your pharmacist whether there is a similar program in your area.

Can natural health products be used by people with diabetes?

There are a number of so-called "natural health products" on the market. It is important to remember, however, that "natural" does not necessarily mean "harmless." In fact, some natural health products can have adverse effects, interact with prescribed drugs, or be contraindicated for various illnesses.

In addition, the quality of natural health products on the market can vary widely, and it is not always possible to know exactly what they contain. An eight-digit natural product number (NPN) identifies products that are authorized for sale in Canada.

People with diabetes who choose to use a natural health product should ask a pharmacist to confirm whether the product is suitable. Doctors should also be informed of the products their patients use.

Can natural health products affect blood glucose levels?

Some natural health products can increase blood glucose, while others can lower it. For example, glucosamine, a supplement used for osteoarthritis, can cause them to rise. Animal studies have also shown that it increases insulin resistance, although the effect of glucosamine on humans appears to be minimal. Because data are limited, however, people who decide to take glucosamine are advised to check their blood glucose regularly to observe the effects. Products that can lower blood glucose include fenugreek, vanadium, bitter melon, gymnema, chromium, American ginseng, and ivy gourd.

It is generally a good idea to talk to a pharmacist or doctor before taking a natural health product to make sure it is both safe and effective. People with diabetes who decide to take a potentially hyperglycemic or hypoglycemic product should take care to check their blood sugar levels more frequently than usual.

According to available information and research, there are currently no natural products recommended to replace antidiabetic drugs or insulin in the treatment of diabetes.

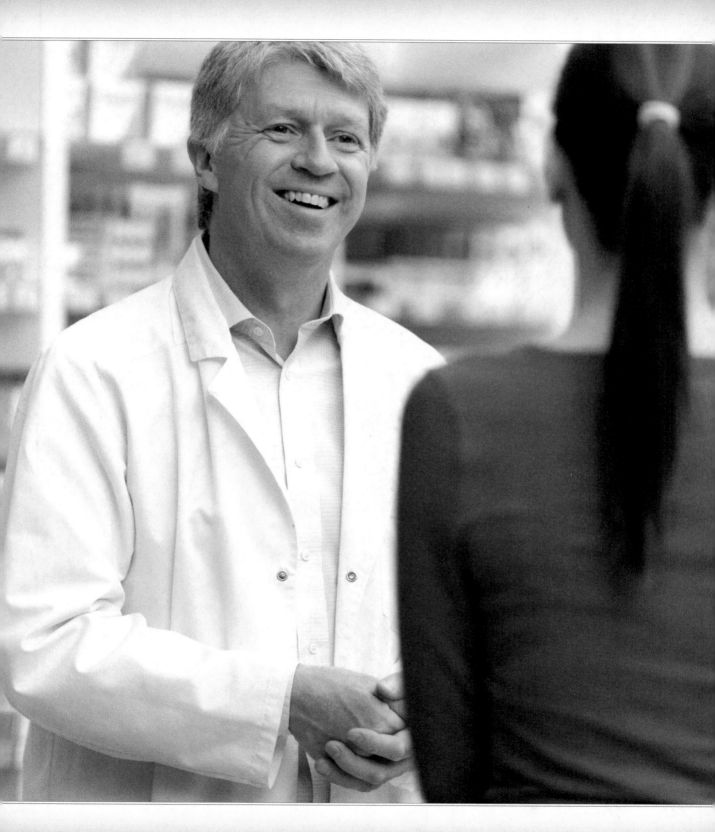

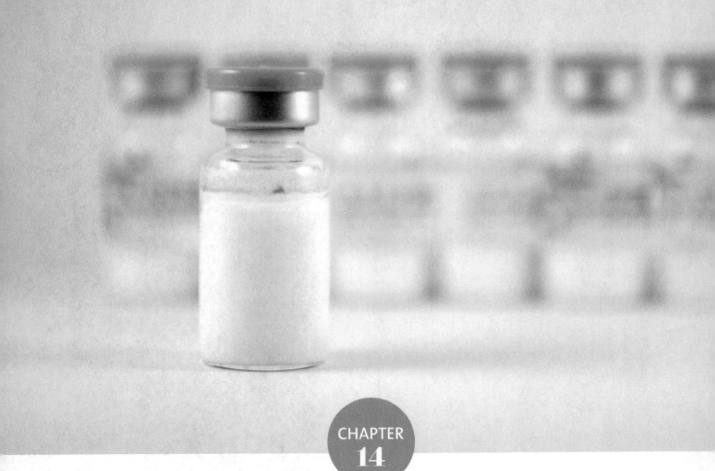

CHAPTER
14

Insulins

What is the role of insulin?

Insulin is a hormone that plays an important role in controlling blood glucose levels. It acts as a kind of "manager," keeping blood glucose down by allowing the sugar in the blood to enter the cells of the body and by telling the liver to lower glucose production.

When is insulin an appropriate treatment for diabetes?

Insulin is routinely used to treat **type 1 diabetes** because this form of the disease is characterized by the inability of the pancreas to produce insulin. It can also be used to treat **type 2 diabetes** if diet, exercise, weight loss and oral or injectable antidiabetic drugs do not control blood glucose sufficiently.

Where does the insulin used for treatment come from?

Insulin is manufactured primarily in laboratories using biogenetic techniques. More specifically, it uses bacteria or yeast that has been genetically programmed to produce insulin.

There are two categories:

1 **Human insulin:** This type is identical to the insulin produced by the pancreas. All insulins with the name Humulin® or Novolin® belong to this category.
2 **Insulin analog:** This type is similar to the insulin produced by the human pancreas, although its structure has been slightly modified to give it new properties. Some examples of this type include Apidra®, Humalog®, NovoRapid,® Humalog® Mix, NovoMix,® Lantus® and Levemir®.

Some types of insulin are of animal origin (purified pork insulin), but they are rarely used. They are mentioned here for informational purposes only.

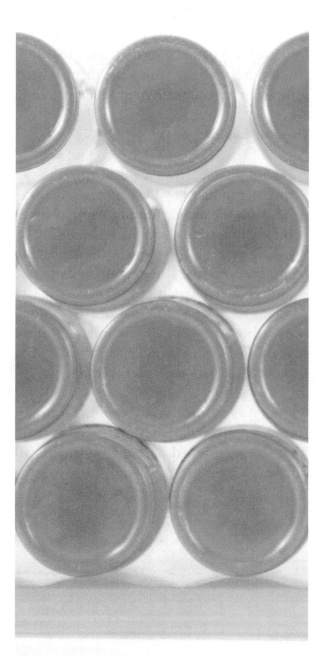

What are the different types of insulin?

The types of insulin are classified according to their action times:

- **onset of action:** the time insulin takes to start working;
- **peak of action:** the time during which the insulin is at maximum effectiveness;
- **duration of action:** the duration of the insulin's effectiveness in the body.

There are six types of insulin:

1 **rapid-acting;**
2 **short-acting;**
3 **intermediate-acting;**
4 **long-acting;**
5 **premixed insulin:** a mixture of **rapid-acting** and **intermediate-acting** insulins;
6 **premixed insulin:** a mixture of **short-acting** and **intermediate-acting** insulins.

What are the action times of the different types of insulin?

TYPES	ONSET OF ACTION	PEAK ACTION	DURATION OF ACTION
Rapid-acting			
• Apidra® (glulisine) • Humalog® (lispro) • NovoRapid ® (aspart)	0 to 15 minutes 0 to 15 minutes 0 to 10 minutes	1 to 1.5 hours 1 to 2 hours 1 to 3 hours	3 to 4 hours 3 to 4 hours 3 to 5 hours
Short-acting (regular)			
• Humulin® R • Novolin® ge Toronto	30 minutes	2 to 4 hours	6 to 8 hours
Intermediate-acting			
• Humulin® N • Novolin® ge NPH	1 to 2 hours	6 to 12 hours	18 to 24 hours
Long-acting			
• Lantus® (glargine) • Levemir® (detemir)	1 hour 1 to 3 hours	Insignificant Insignificant	24 hours 20 to 24 hours
Premixed rapid-acting and intermediate-acting			
• Humalog® Mix 25* • Humalog® Mix 50*	0 to 15 minutes	1 to 2 hours and 6 to 12 hours	18 to 24 hours
• NovoMix® 30**	10 to 20 minutes	1 to 4 hours	Up to 24 hours
Premixed short-acting and intermediate acting*			
• Humulin® 30/70 • Novolin® ge 30/70 • Novolin® ge 40/60 • Novolin® ge 50/50	30 minutes	2 to 4 hours and 6 to 12 hours	18 to 24 hours

* Humalog® Mix 25 is a mixture of 25% lispro insulin (rapid-acting insulin) and 75% lispro protamine insulin (intermediate-acting insulin).
Humalog® Mix 50 is a 50%-50% mixture of these two types of insulin.

** NovoMix® 30 is a mixture of 30% insulin aspart (rapid-acting insulin) and 70% insulin aspart protamine (intermediate-acting insulin)

***The first number corresponds to the percentage of short-acting insulin and the second to the percentage of intermediate-acting NPH insulin.

Note: The values indicated in the table may vary from one individual to another.

RAPID-ACTING INSULIN

Action time

Onset	Peak	Duration
0 - 15 min	1 - 3 hours	3 - 5 hours

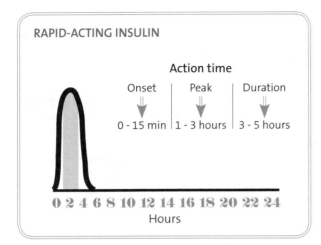

Hours

SHORT-ACTING INSULIN

Action time

Onset	Peak	Duration
30 min	2 - 4 hours	6 - 8 hours

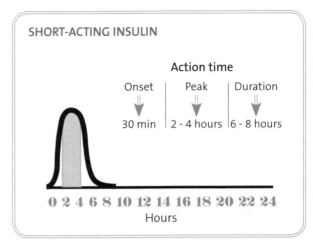

Hours

INTERMEDIATE-ACTING INSULIN

Action time

Onset	Peak	Duration
1 - 2 hours	6 - 12 hours	18 - 24 hours

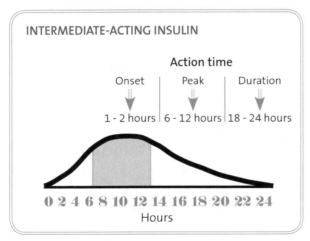

Hours

LONG-ACTING INSULIN

Action time

Onset	Peak	Duration
1 hour	None	24 hours

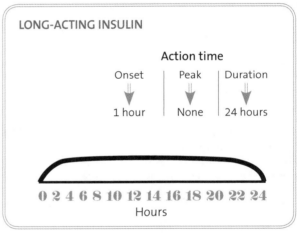

Hours

PREMIXED RAPID- AND INTERMEDIATE-ACTING INSULIN

Action time

Onset	Peak	Duration
0 - 15 min	1 - 2 hours and 6 - 12 hours	18 - 24 hours

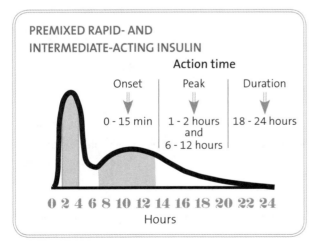

Hours

PREMIXED SHORT- AND INTERMEDIATE-ACTING INSULIN

Action time

Onset	Peak	Duration
30 min	2 - 4 hours and 6 - 12 hours	18 - 24 hours

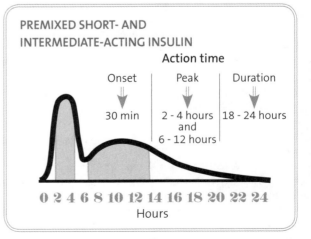

Hours

What roles do the different types of insulin play?

Rapid-acting and short-acting insulins are used primarily to control blood sugar at mealtimes. Intermediate-acting and long-acting insulins are used to control blood sugar during fasting periods, which are generally between meals and overnight.

How many insulin injections are required daily?

In general, insulin therapy requires from one to four injections daily. The number and timing of injections as well as the types of insulin vary from one individual to another, and treatment is adapted to the person's lifestyle. The goal is to maintain blood glucose as close as possible to normal levels.

What are the most frequently prescribed insulin regimens?

There are several insulin regimens. Here are four of the most frequently prescribed:

1 The "basal-prandial" regimen involves the injection of rapid-acting or short-acting insulin before each meal and intermediate-acting or long-acting basal insulin at bedtime. Although basal insulin is usually administered in one injection, it can also be given in several injections throughout the day. The dose of rapid-acting or short-acting insulin can be fixed (fixed carbohydrate regimen) or correspond to the amount of carbohydrates consumed in the meal (variable carbohydrate regimen). The variable carbohydrate regimen is almost exclusively prescribed with rapid-acting insulin. In a variable carbohydrate diet, the dose is expressed as a ratio, for example, 1 unit/10 g of carbohydrates (1 unit of insulin for every 10 g of carbohydrates consumed).

2 The "split-mixed" regimen involves the injection of intermediate-acting and either rapid- or short-acting insulin before breakfast and dinner. The pre-dinner injection of intermediate-acting insulin is sometimes postponed to bedtime to control glucose levels overnight and to help prevent nocturnal hypoglycemia.

3 The "premixed" regimen involves the injection of a mixed dose of rapid-acting or short-acting insulin and intermediate-acting insulin before breakfast and dinner.

4 The "**combined**" regimen involves the injection of intermediate-acting or long-acting insulin at bedtime and antidiabetic medications during the day.

What is intensive insulin therapy?

Intensive insulin therapy consists of multiple insulin injections (for example, the "basal-prandial" regimen) or the use of an insulin pump combined with the monitoring of blood glucose and self-adjusted insulin doses. People following this regimen must learn to calculate the amount of carbohydrates in their meals to adjust their doses, which is expressed as a ratio (e.g. x units/10 g of carbohydrates) and based on the amount of carbohydrates consumed. This therapy tries to mimic the normal release of insulin from the pancreas. The goal is to maintain blood glucose levels as close to normal as possible.

How much insulin is required to control blood glucose?

Insulin doses are initially determined by the doctor and then vary according to blood glucose readings. Doses are measured in **units**. Some people inject fixed doses while others calculate their doses according to the carbohydrate content of their meals. Whatever the regimen, doses should be regularly modified according to factors such as diet, exercise, and illness.

How should insulin injections be timed in relation to meals and bedtime?

MEALS:

- **Rapid-acting insulin** should be injected **just before meals** (or in the case of Apidra® and Humalog®, no more than 15 minutes before and in the case of NovoRapid®, no more than 10 minutes before), whether or not the insulin is premixed.
- **Short-acting insulin** should be injected **15 to 30 minutes before meals**, whether or not it is premixed.

This allows the peak action of the insulin to coincide with the peak absorption of the carbohydrates consumed.

BEDTIME:

- **Intermediate-acting or long-acting insulin** is generally injected at approximately 10 p.m. The time of injection should be as regular as possible.

This allows the peak action time of intermediate-acting insulin to coincide with breakfast.

OPTIMAL INSULIN INJECTION TIME	
Insulin	**Optimal injection time**
Apidra® Humalog® NovoRapid® Humalog® Mix 25 ou 50 NovoMix® 30	• Immediately before meals (a maximum of 10 minutes before for NovoRapid® and NovoMix® and a maximum of 15 minutes before for Apidra® and Humalog®) • May be administered immediately after meals (e.g., in the case of variable appetite and unpredictable dietary intake)
Humulin® R Novolin® ge Toronto Humulin® 30/70 Novolin® ge 30/70, 40/60, 50/50	• 15 to 30 minutes before meals
Humulin® N Novolin® ge NPH	• If at bedtime: always at the same time, usually around 10:00 p.m. • If at breakfast or supper: at the same time as the rapid-acting or short-acting insulin
Lantus® Levemir®	• Always at the same time, usually at bedtime, around 10 p.m. • If twice a day: morning and bedtime or at dinner

What is the most common adverse effect of insulin therapy?

Hypoglycemia is the most common adverse effect seen in people taking insulin. The risk of hypoglycemia is much higher when insulin action is at its peak. Being well-informed about insulin and the rules governing dosage adjustment can lower the risk.

How should insulin be used to effectively control diabetes?

To control diabetes with insulin injections, it is important to:
- closely follow your meal plan;
- check blood glucose levels regularly;
- be well-informed about the insulin you use; and
- self-adjust your insulin doses after receiving the necessary training from your health care team.

What time of day should a person with diabetes who is taking insulin check blood glucose?

A person with diabetes on insulin therapy should measure blood glucose **before meals and at bedtime (before a snack).** It is also helpful to occasionally measure blood glucose after meals (one or two hours after the first mouthful) or during the night (around 2 a.m.) to check for nocturnal hypoglycemia. If the person is sick, blood glucose measurements should be taken more often. It should also be measured every time the person feels discomfort that could indicate hypoglycemia or hyperglycemia. The frequency and time of day of the checks should be adapted to the treatment being followed (e.g., number of injections per day), the information needed to make adjustments, and the clinical situation.

MAIN INSULIN REGIMENS

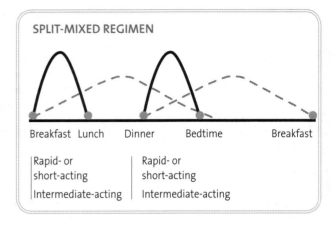

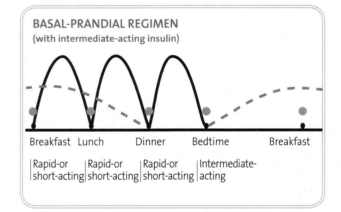

BASAL-PRANDIAL REGIMEN (with long acting insulin)

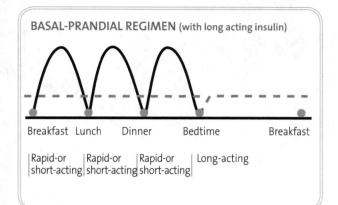

Breakfast Lunch   Dinner   Bedtime   Breakfast

| Rapid-or | Rapid-or | Rapid-or | Long-acting |
| short-acting | short-acting | short-acting | |

PREMIXED REGIMEN

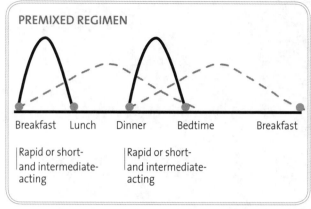

Breakfast   Lunch   Dinner   Bedtime   Breakfast

Rapid or short-	Rapid or short-
and intermediate-	and intermediate-
acting	acting

COMBINED REGIMEN

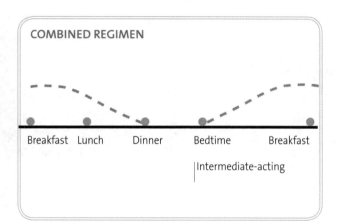

Breakfast Lunch   Dinner   Bedtime   Breakfast

| Intermediate-acting |

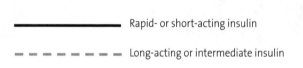

Rapid- or short-acting insulin

Long-acting or intermediate insulin

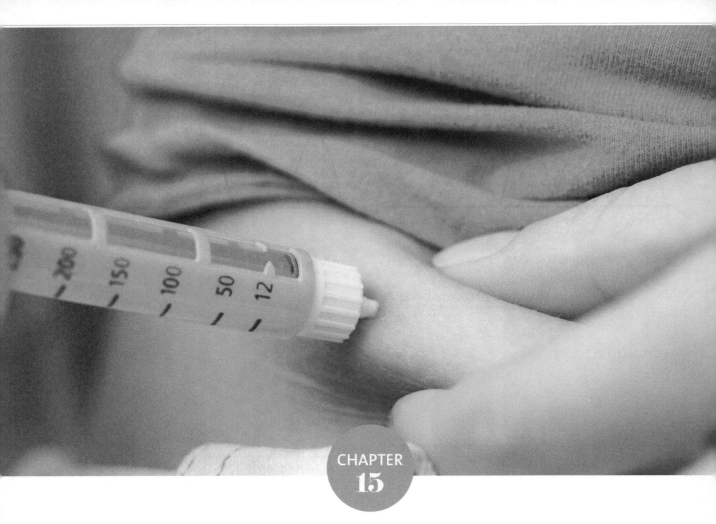

Preparing and Injecting Insulin

What devices are used to inject insulin?

Three types of devices are used in inject insulin:

- **Syringe:** Syringes consists of a cylinder and a plunger fitted with a fine needle. Syringes come in different volumes: 100 units, 50 units or 30 units. The finer the needle, the greater the gauge (for instance, a 30-gauge needle is finer than a 29-gauge needle). Also, the finer the needle, the shorter it is (6 mm as opposed to 12.7 mm). **Use of the 6 mm needle (the shortest) is encouraged.** Syringes also come with different scale graduations (½ unit, 1 unit and 2 units).
- **Pen device:** This device is slightly larger than a pen and has three parts: the cap, which covers the pen, the cartridge-holder, which contains the insulin cartridge, and the body, which contains the plunger. A dial lets you select the desired dose.
- **Insulin pump:** This device, approximately the size of a cell phone, continuously releases rapid-acting insulin by means of a cannula (thin tube) or pod. The cannula is inserted under the skin with a small needle that is then removed. When the pod is used, the insertion mechanism is automatic. Tubes and pods must be changed every two or three days.

How do I prepare and inject a single type of insulin with a syringe?

There are three steps to preparing and injecting a single type of insulin with a syringe.

Prepare the material

1 **Wash your hands** with soap and water and dry them well.
2 Lay out the **material:** syringe, insulin vial, alcohol swab, cotton ball.
   - Use a new syringe for each injection.
   - Use a vial of insulin at room temperature.
3 Check the label on the vial to make sure you have the right **type of insulin.**
4 Check the **expiry dates** on the label. Check the date printed by the manufacturer and the date recorded when the vial was opened (*see in chapter 17 the table listing the temperatures and maximum storage times recommended by insulin manufacturers*).

Do not prepare syringes in advance if you are using Lantus® (glargine) insulin because it will become cloudy. Levemir® (detemir) and Apidra® (glulisine) also should not be prepared in advance because of a lack of information about its stability.

Draw up the insulin

1 If the **contents are opaque**, roll the vial between your hands and turn it upside down to mix the suspension thoroughly (do not shake). Place the vial upright on the table.

2 **Clean the cap** of the vial with the alcohol swab.

3 **Pull back the plunger** of the syringe to draw up an amount of air equal to the amount of insulin to be injected.

4 **Insert the needle** into the rubber cap of the insulin vial.

5 **Inject the air** into the vial.

6 **Turn the vial and syringe** upside down.

7 **Pull the plunger back slowly** to draw up the number of insulin units to be injected.

- Make sure there are no air bubbles in the syringe; bubbles can prevent the full amount of insulin from being injected.
- Push and pull the plunger until any air bubbles disappear.
- Check the syringe to make sure no insulin has been lost; if there has, repeat this step.

Inject the insulin and record the data

1 **Choose the injection site.**
Avoid injecting insulin into a limb or part of the body used for any planned physical activity (for example, a thigh if you intend to take a walk, an arm if you intend to play tennis, etc.).

2 **Choose the injection point** in the site, paying attention to the condition of the skin.
Avoid any crease, bump, growth, bruise, blotch or painful spot.

3 **Wash the skin** with soapy water, rinse, and let dry.
Make sure the injection point is clean. The use of alcohol at home is optional.

4 Depending on the length of the needle:
- **6 mm:** Do not inject into a skin lift.
- **8 mm:** Inject into a skin lift. Delicately lift the skin with your thumb and index finger, taking care not to lift the muscle tissue, and maintain the lift until the end of the injection.
- Needles longer than 8 mm are not recommended.

5 Hold the syringe like a pencil and **pierce the skin.**
Inject the insulin into the subcutaneous tissue (under the skin).

6 **Inject all the insulin,** pushing the plunger all the way down.
- **Do not pull the plunger back:** Raising the plunger to check whether the injection is at the right spot can damage the skin.
- Leave the needle in place for about 5 seconds.

7 **Withdraw the needle** and carefully press the cotton ball to the injection point.

8 **Dispose of the needle** safely in an approved medical waste container.

9 **Record the number of insulin units** and the type of insulin injected in the appropriate column of your self-monitoring logbook

Are any precautions necessary when mixing two types of insulin in the same syringe?

When mixing clear and opaque insulin in the same syringe, certain precautions are necessary:

- Avoid contaminating a vial of one type of insulin with another type. The recommended order for drawing up insulin may vary from one diabetes clinic to another. Some clinics recommend drawing up clear, rapid-acting insulin (Apidra®, Humalog® or NovoRapid®) or fast-acting insulin (Humulin® R or Novolin® ge Toronto) before opaque (Humulin® N or Novolin® ge NPH). **Other clinics advise drawing up opaque insulin before clear so that any contamination of the clear by the opaque can be easily detected.**
- If one insulin is contaminated by another, the contaminated vial must be discarded because its action time (start, peak, duration) might be modified. Cross-contamination of insulins can hamper blood glucose control.
- Be sure to draw up the insulins in the same order every time; this will help you avoid errors.

- It is generally recommended to avoid mixing insulins from different manufacturers in the same syringe.
- **Never mix Lantus® (glargine) and Levemir® (detemir) insulins with another type of insulin.**

How do I prepare and inject two types of insulin with the same syringe?

There are three steps to preparing and injecting two types of insulin with the same syringe.

Prepare the material

1 **Wash your hands** with soap and water and dry them well.

2 **Lay out the material:** syringe, insulin vials, alcohol swab, cotton ball.
- Use a new syringe for each injection.
- Use vials of insulin stored at room temperature.

3 Check the labels of the vials to make sure you have the **right types of insulin**.

4 Check the **expiry dates** on the labels. Check the date printed by the manufacturer and the date recorded when the vials were opened (*see the table in chapter 17 on page 156 listing the temperature and maximum storage times recommended by insulin manufacturers*).

Draw up the insulins

The recommended order for drawing up the insulins may vary from one diabetes clinic to another.

1 **Roll the vial of opaque insulin** between your hands and turn it upside down to mix the suspension thoroughly (**do not shake**). Place the vial upright on the table.

2 **Clean the caps** of the vials of opaque insulin and clear insulin with an alcohol swab.

3 **Inject air into the vial of clear insulin.**
Pull back the plunger of the syringe to draw in an amount of air equal to the amount of clear insulin to be injected. Insert the needle into the rubber cap of the clear insulin vial. Inject the air into the vial. Do not touch the insulin or draw any up. Withdraw the needle from the vial.

4 **Inject air into the vial of opaque insulin.**
Pull back the plunger of the syringe to draw in an amount of air equal to the amount of opaque insulin to be injected. Insert the needle into the rubber cap of the opaque insulin vial and inject the air into the vial. Leave the needle in the vial.

5 **Draw up the required dose of opaque insulin.**
- Turn the opaque insulin vial and the needle upside down. Pull the plunger back slowly to draw up the number of units of opaque insulin to be injected.
- Withdraw the needle from the vial.
- Make sure there are no air bubbles in the syringe; bubbles may prevent the full amount of insulin from being injected.
- Push and pull the plunger until the bubbles disappear.

- Check the syringe to make sure no insulin has been lost; if there has, repeat this step.

6 **Draw up the required dose of clear insulin.**
Turn the clear insulin vial upside down. Insert the needle into the rubber cap of the clear insulin vial. Do not allow any opaque insulin to enter the clear insulin vial. Pull the plunger back slowly to draw up the number of units of clear insulin to be injected. Withdraw the needle from the vial.

If you have drawn up too much clear insulin:
- **discard** the insulin drawn up, but save the syringe;
- **start the process again**, from the beginning.

If the vial of clear insulin is contaminated by opaque insulin:
- **discard** the vial of clear insulin;
- **start** the process again from the beginning with a new vial.

Inject the insulins and record the data

1 **Choose the injection site.**

   Avoid injecting insulin into a limb or part of the body used for any planned physical activity (for example, a thigh if you intend to take a walk, an arm if you intend to play tennis, etc.).

2 **Choose the injection point in the injection site,** paying attention to the condition of the skin.

   Avoid any crease, bump, growth, bruise, blotch or painful spot.

3 **Wash the skin** with soapy water, rinse, and let dry.

   Make sure the injection point is clean. The use of alcohol at home is optional.

4 **Depending on the length of the needle:**
   - **6 mm:** Do not inject into a skin lift.
   - **8 mm:** Inject into a skin lift. Delicately lift the skin with your thumb and index finger, taking care not to lift the muscle tissue, and maintain the lift until the end of the injection.
   - Needles longer than 8 mm are not recommended.

5 Hold the syringe like a pencil and **pierce the skin.**

   Inject the insulin into the subcutaneous tissue (under the skin).

6 **Inject all of the insulin,** pushing the plunger all the way down.
   - **Do not pull the plunger back:** Raising the plunger to check whether the injection is at the right spot can damage the skin.
   - **Leave the needle in place** for about 5 seconds.

7 **Withdraw the needle** and carefully press the cotton ball to the injection point.

8 **Dispose of the syringe safely** in an approved medical waste container.

9 **Record the number of insulin units** and the type of insulin injected in the appropriate column of your self-monitoring logbook.

What types of pen devices are currently available?

Several models of pen devices are available (list revised on May 1, 2013):

Pen device	Manufacturer	Cartridge	Graduation	Dosage dial
HumaPen Luxura ® HD	Eli Lilly Canada Inc.	3 mL	0.5 units at a time	0.5 to 30 units
HumaPen Luxura®	Eli Lilly Canada Inc.	3 mL	1 unit at a time	1 to 60 units
HumaPen Savvio®	Eli Lilly Canada Inc.	3 mL	1 unit at a time	1 to 60 units
HumaLog KwikPen® (pre-filled)	Eli Lilly Canada Inc.	3 mL	1 unit at a time	1 to 60 units
Humulin®R KwikPen® (pre-filled)	Eli Lilly Canada Inc.	3 mL	1 unit at a time	1 to 60 units
HumalogMix25® KwikPen® (pre-filled)	Eli Lilly Canada Inc.	3 mL	1 unit at a time	1 to 60 units
HumalogMix50 KwikPen® (pre-filled)	Eli Lilly Canada Inc.	3 mL	1 unit at a time	1 to 60 units
Humulin®N KwikPen® (pre-filled)	Eli Lilly Canada Inc.	3 mL	1 unit at a time	1 to 60 units
NovoPen Echo®	Novo Nordisk Canada Inc.	3 mL	0.5 units at a time	0.5 to 0 units
Novo-Pen® 4	Novo Nordisk Canada Inc.	3 mL	1 unit at a time	1 to 60 units
NovoRapid® FlexTouch® (pre-filled)	Novo Nordisk Canada Inc.	3 mL	1 unit at a time	1 to 80 units
ClikSTAR®	sanofi-aventis Canada Inc.	3 mL	1 unit at a time	1 to 80 units
Apidra® SoloSTAR® (pre-filled)	sanofi-aventis Canada Inc.	3 mL	1 unit at a time	1 to 80 units
Lantus® SoloSTAR® (pre-filled)	sanofi-aventis Canada Inc.	3 mL	1 unit at a time	1 to 80 units

Check the product monograph for the type of insulin and the type of needle that can be used with the selected pen device. If using two types of insulin that are not premixed, use two different pen devices.

Are there any other products useful for the treatment of diabetes?

Yes. There are a number of products on the market made specifically to help people with diabetes. For example:

Frio® coolers

Cases to protect insulin from excessive heat. Talk to a pharmacist (www.diabetesexpress.ca or 1 866 418-3392)

i-Port™ Advance, 6 mm or 9 mm

Device with a discreet injection port with an inserter. Once in place, it can be used for three days to inject insulin. (Patton Medical Devices, www.i-port.com or 1 877 763-7678).

INJEX 30

Needle-free injection system using pressure to propel a fine stream of insulin through the skin (INJEX PHARMA AG, www.injex.ca or 1 855 823-5533).

How do I prepare and inject insulin with a pen device?

There are three steps to preparing and injecting insulin with a pen device.

Prepare the material

1 **Wash your hands** with soap and water and dry them well.
2 Lay out the **material**: pen device, insulin cartridge, needle, alcohol swab.
   - Use a new needle for each injection.
   - Use an insulin cartridge stored at room temperature.
3 Check the **type of insulin and the quantity of insulin** remaining in the cartridge.
4 Check the **expiry dates** on the label. Check the date printed by the manufacturer and the date recorded when the cartridges were opened (*see the table in chapter 17 on page 156 listing the temperature and maximum storage times recommended by insulin manufacturers*).
   - Do not refrigerate the pen device; cold temperatures can damage it or cause air bubbles to form in the cartridge.
   - Do not share your pen device with anyone else.

Select a dose of insulin

1 **Bring opaque insulin to a uniform appearance.** Roll the pen between your palms about ten times to loosen the insulin from the sides, then turn the pen device over the same number of times. There is a glass marble inside the opaque insulin cartridge that slides from one end to the other to mix the insulin. Do not shake the pen vigorously, as this can damage the insulin and reduce its effectiveness.

2 **Screw the needle onto the pen and fill up the empty space in the needle,** selecting one unit of insulin at a time until a drop of insulin appears at the tip of the needle when pointed upwards.

3 **Select the insulin dose** by turning the dosage ring to the desired number of units.

Inject the insulin and record the data

1 **Choose the injection site.** Avoid injecting insulin into a limb or part of the body used for any planned physical activity (for example, a thigh if you intend to take a walk, an arm if you intend to play tennis, etc.).

2 **Choose the injection point** in the site, paying attention to the condition of the skin. Avoid any crease, bump, growth, bruise, blotch or painful spot.

3 **Clean the skin** with an alcohol swab and let it dry. Make sure the injection point is clean. The use of alcohol at home is optional.

4 The use of needles shorter than **4, 5, or 6 mm** are encouraged, since they generally do not require a skin lift for injection.

5 When using **8 mm** needles, a skin lift must be maintained until the end of the injection.
   - Delicately lift the skin with your thumb and index finger, taking care not to lift the muscle tissue.
   - Needles longer than 8 mm are not recommended.

6 Hold the pen device like a pencil and **pierce the skin.** Inject the insulin into the subcutaneous tissue (under the skin).

7 **Inject all of the insulin,** pushing the plunger all the way down. **Leave the needle in place** for about **10 seconds** or longer for larger doses.

8 **Withdraw the needle** and carefully press the cotton ball to the injection point. **Remove** the needle from the pen device when the injection is complete. Discard the needle safely in an approved medical waste container.

9 **Record the number of insulin units** and the type of insulin injected in the appropriate column of your self-monitoring logbook.

What are the recommended insulin injection techniques?

Insulin must be injected into subcutaneous tissue (under the skin).

1 Needles of 4, 5, and 6 mm are appropriate for anyone with diabetes, regardless of their body mass (BMI). Clinical research does not support the recommendation of needles longer than 8 mm.

2 Your insulin injection technique should be personalized and chosen with the help of a health professional.

3 Several factors must be considered, including age (child or adult) and weight (thin or obese). The length of the needle, the need for a skin lift, and the angle of injection can vary from person to person.

- Most people can reach subcutaneous tissue by injecting at a 90° angle.
- Thin people or children may need to perform a skin lift, use short needles, or inject at a 45º angle to avoid injecting into muscle tissue.

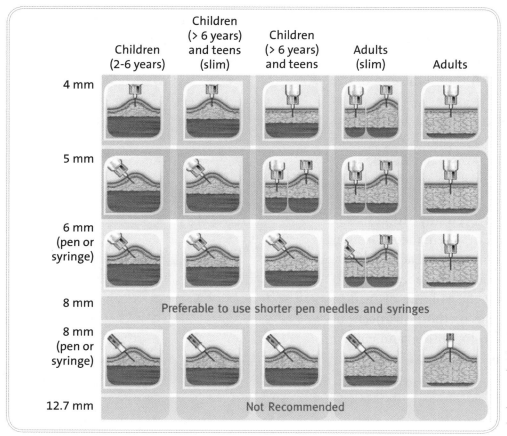

From "Educational tools based on FIT Canada's Recommendations for Best Practice in Injection Technique," Fit Technique Plus, Technique for All, 2013. www.fit4diabetes.com

4 Using a new needle for each injection can reduce the risk of needles breaking in the skin, blocked needles, lipohypertrophy (bump at the injection point), inadequate dosage, and indirect harm (e.g., abcess).

- When the injection is subcutaneous, the tissue under the skin appears normal.
- Blood or bruising at the injection point may indicate that a small capillary has been penetrated, although this will not affect the absorption of insulin.
- A **white site** appearing when the needle is withdrawn can indicate that the insulin has not been injected deeply enough.
- When the technique requires injection into a skin lift, delicately lift the skin between your thumb and index finger, taking care not to lift any muscle tissue, and maintain the lift until the end of the injection.
- Blood glucose levels must be checked more carefully if a change is made from a long needle to a short needle. Be sure that insulin absorption remains at the same level.

5 There have not yet been any studies concerning the maximum subcutaneous insulin dose that can be administered at one point. Several factors have to be taken into account, including the volume of insulin injected at once, the method of injection, the speed of insulin absorption, and pain at the injection point.

- In some cases it is recommended that doses of 50 units or more be distributed between two injection points to make absorption easier. A new needle should be used for each injection.
- One of the factors affecting the speed of subcutaneous insulin absorption is the volume injected. The greater the volume of insulin, the more slowly it is absorbed, and the longer it will take before absorption begins.
- Large amounts of insulin are often associated with a loss of insulin on the skin surface.
- Studies have shown that in most cases, pain at the injection point increases when the volume injected is greater than 50 units.

What should be done with used prefilled pen devices, syringes, needles and lancets?

A system to dispose of used prefilled disposable pen devices, syringes, needles and lancets has been implemented to ensure that these items are not left in inappropriate places and cause accidents. All needles should be disposed of safely, in an approved medical waste container.

Special containers can be obtained **for free** in pharmacies and community health clinics. Once filled, the container can be brought to one of four places for disposal: a pharmacy, a community health clinic, a diabetes clinic or a participating community organization. If no special containers are available, place the used material in a safely sealed plastic container for disposal. **Needles should never be re-sheathed.**

What are the recommendations for the use of safety devices in the treatment of diabetes?

In Canada, it is estimated that more than 70,000 people injure themselves on syringes every year.

- It is essential for administrators of health establishments to develop and implement safe work practices.
- It is recommended that health professionals and other individuals involved in medical treatment use safety engineered devices with built-in safety mechanisms.
- Safety engineered devices should also be used at home in any situation that presents a heightened risk of cross-contamination.

www.fit4diabetes.com
FIT Canada. Berard, L., Desrochers, F., Husband, Al., MacNeill, G., Roscoe, R. Forum for Injection Technique. "Recommendations for Best Practices in Injection Technique," 2012. 1–26.

FIT Technique Plus. Technique for All, 2013. Educational tools based on FIT Canada "Recommendations for Best practices in Injection Techhnique," 2012.

FIT4Safety Caanda. MacNeill, G., Berard, L., Arsenault, J., DeCiantis, K., Dudziak, S., Trimble, L.A., Koropas, S. "Recommendations for Best Practice in the Safe Use of Diabetes Medical Waste," 2013. 1–14.

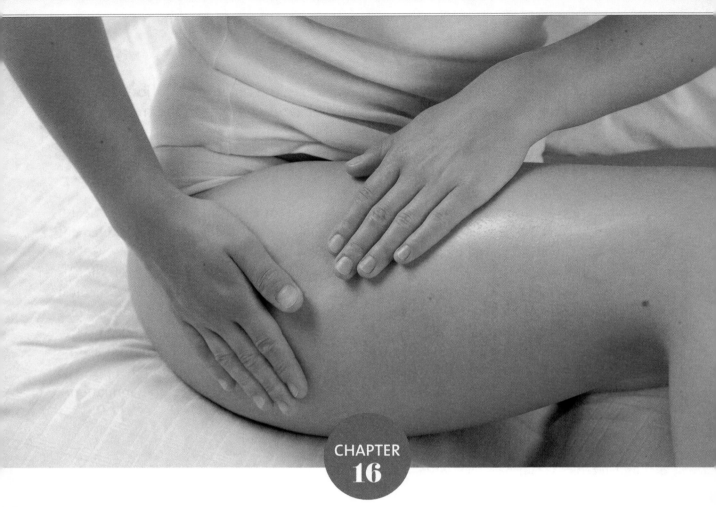

CHAPTER
16

Insulin Injection: Injection Site Rotation

What parts of the body are the best places to inject insulin?

Insulin can be injected in different parts of the body. There are eight standard injection sites:

Sites 1 and 2	**Abdomen:** right and left sides, except for 3.5 cm (2 fingers) around the navel
Sites 3 and 4	**Arms:** antero-external (outer front) surface
Sites 5 and 6	**Thighs:** antero-external (outer front) surface
Sites 7 and 8	**Buttocks:** fleshy upper parts

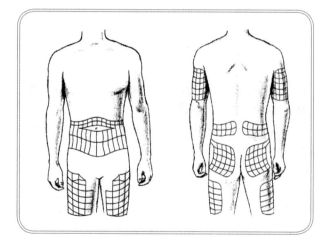

Unless it is possible to perform a skin fold, injecting into the distended abdomen of a pregnant woman can damage the skin and is not recommended.

How many injection points are there in each site?

Within each **injection site**, there are multiple **injection points**. The entire surface of a site can be used, as long as the same injection point is not used more than **once a month**.

What distance should there be between injection points within the same site?

Within the same site, each injection point should be 2 to 3 cm (2 fingers) from the point of the previous injection:

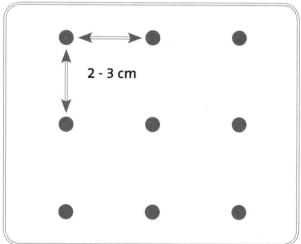

Injection points

Why is a structured rotation of injection sites and points recommended?

Injection points should be rotated for **each insulin injection** to prevent **lipodystrophy** (bumps or indentations from repeated injections at the same point). Not only are these subcutaneous deformations unattractive, more importantly, they hamper the absorption of insulin and the proper blood glucose control.

People with diabetes should be taught a personalized structured rotation for their injection sites and points.

Here is an example of a structured rotation for the abdomen and thighs:

- Divide the injection sites into sections (quadrants or halves).
- Use one section per week, rotating either clockwise or counter-clockwise within it, eventually using the entire site

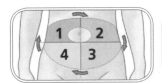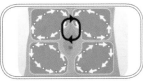

From FIT Canada, FIT Canada. Berard, L., Desrochers, F., Husband, Al., MacNeill, G., Roscoe, R. Forum for Injection Technique, "Recommendations for Best Practice in Injection Technique," 1-26, 2012

Does the injection site have an impact on the absorption of the insulin injected?

Yes. The speed of absorption of any one type of insulin varies according to the injection site used.

- Insulin is absorbed **fastest** from the **abdomen**, followed by the arms, thighs and buttocks, in that order.
- **Speed of absorption:**
  abdomen > arms > thighs > buttocks
  (> : greater than)
- **The abdomen is the region where absorption is the most constant.**

What other factors influence the speed of insulin absorption?

Intense exercise increases the rate of absorption if insulin is injected into the part of the body being exercised.

- For example, insulin injected into your thigh is absorbed more quickly if you take a walk or play tennis afterwards.

Other factors such as heat (e.g., from the sun, in a bath), the depth of the injection, or massage at the point can affect the speed of absorption.

How can the amount of insulin absorbed be maintained at a stable level regardless of the injection site used?

To ensure that the amount of insulin absorbed varies as little as possible regardless of the injection site being used, do the following:

1 **Prevent lipodystrophy by:**
- changing the injection point every time;
- following a structured rotation, dividing injection sites into sections;
- examine and palpate injection sites when standing, looking for bumps, lumps, or dents;
- change needles for every injection;
- inform your doctor if a skin reaction (indentation) occurs at the injection point after administering an injectable antidiabetic drug.

2 Inject rapid-acting and short-acting insulin into the abdomen, either alone or mixed with intermediate-acting insulin. Change the injection point each time.

3 **The arm is generally not recommended for self-injection because the site may be difficult to reach and this may cause an increased risk of intramuscular injection.**

4 Inject intermediate-acting or long-acting insulin not mixed with rapid-acting or short-acting insulin into the **thigh or buttocks** to ensure the slowest possible absorption.

5 If several insulin injections are administered at different times of the day, the same injection site should be used at the same time every day.

6 A particular site (taking into account speed of absorption) should be used for a given insulin (taking into account time of action) according to the time of injection (taking into account current activity).

7 Lantus® (glargine) and Levemir® (detemir) insulins are long-acting and can generally meet basal insulin needs with one daily injection. Sometimes two injections are necessary. These insulins are usually injected in sites of slow absorption such as the thigh, **although the speed of absorption of Lantus® is similar in every site of injection.**

IN SUMMARY:

TYPES OF INSULIN	SUGGESTED INJECTION SITES	
	Abdomen	Thighs and buttocks
Rapid or short-acting	Preferable	---
Rapid-acting or mixed short- and intermediate-acting	Preferable	---
Intermediate-acting alone	---	Preferable
Long-acting	---	Preferable

1 FIT Canada. Berard, L., Desrochers, F., Husband, Al., MacNeill, G., Roscoe, R. Forum for Injection Technique. "Recommendations for Best Practice in Injection Technique," 1-26, 2012

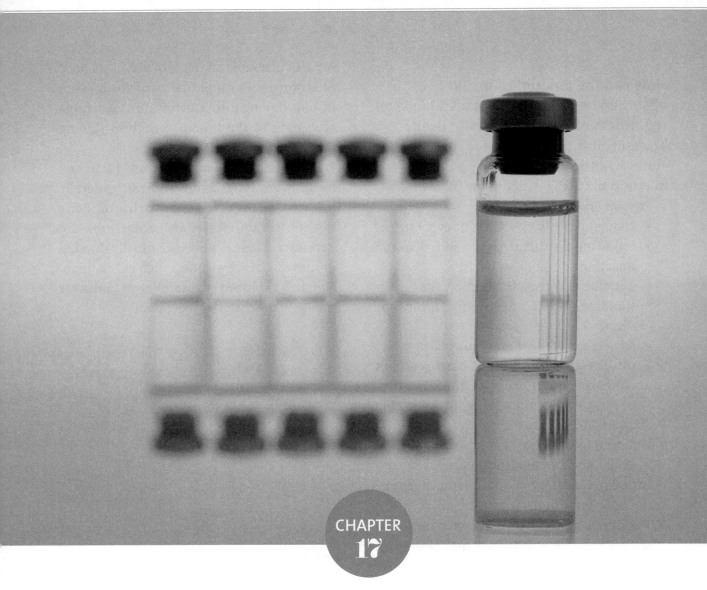

Storing Insulin

Why should precautions be taken when storing insulin?

Insulin is fragile. To ensure that your insulin preserve their effectiveness, follow the manufacturer's recommendations for storage. Using improperly stored insulin can impair blood glucose control.

What precautions should be taken when storing insulin?

- Insulin that is **currently in use** can be stored for up to **one month at room temperature**. Injecting cold insulin can cause pain at the injection site.
- **Reserve supplies** of insulin should be kept in the **refrigerator**. If stored this way, the insulin will remain usable until the expiry date indicated by the manufacturer.
- Insulin should never be exposed to direct sunlight or heat. Although the product will not necessarily change in appearance, it must nevertheless be discarded if it's been exposed to excessive heat.
- Insulin should never be frozen. Again, the product will not necessarily change in appearance, but insulin that has been frozen must be discarded.
- Pen injectors should not be stored in the refrigerator, since the cold can damage them or create air bubbles in the cartridge. Reserve supplies of insulin already preloaded in disposable pens, however, should be refrigerated.
- Spare insulin syringes that have been prepared in advance should be kept in the refrigerator in an upright or slightly slanted position, with the needle (and its cap) pointing upwards. This will prevent insulin particles from clogging the needle.
- The date the vial, cartridge or pen injector was opened should be recorded.
- There should always be a reserve of insulin in the refrigerator for an emergency (breakage, for example).

What are the specific recommendations for storing insulin?

The following table shows the temperatures and storage times recommended by insulin manufacturers, listed by brand and format.

FORMAT	BRANDS	RECOMMENDED TEMPERATURE	MAXIMUM STORAGE
Unopened vial or cartridge	Apidra® Humalog® Humulin® Lantus® Levemir®	2°C – 8°C	Expiry date on container
	Novolin® NovoRapid® NovoMix®	2°C – 10°C	Expiry date on container
Opened vial	Apidra® Humulin® Novolin®	Room temperature Maximum 25°C	28 days
	Humalog® NovoRapid® Lantus®	Room temperature Maximum 30°C	28 days
Opened cartridge	Apidra® Humulin®	Room temperature Maximum 25°C	28 days
	Humalog® Humalog® Mix Novolin® NovoRapid® NovoMix® Lantus®	Room temperature Maximum 30°C	28 days
	Levemir®	Room temperature Maximum 30°C	42 days

FORMAT	BRANDS	RECOMMENDED TEMPERATURE	MAXIMUM STORAGE
Reserve supply of disposable prefilled pen devices	Apidra® SoloSTAR® Humalog® KwikPen® Humalog® Mix KwikPen® Humulin® N KwikPen® Humulin® R KwikPen® Lantus® SoloSTAR®	2°C – 8°C	Expiry date on container
	NovoRapid® FlexTouch®	2°C – 10°C	Expiry date on container
Opened disposable prefilled pen devices	Apidra® SoloSTAR® Humulin® N KwikPen® Humulin® R KwikPen®	Room temperature Maximum 25°C	28 days
	Humalog® KwikPen® Humalog® Mix KwikPen® NovoRapid® FlexTouch® Lantus® SoloSTAR®	Room temperature Maximum 30°C	28 days
Pre-prepared syringe*	Humulin® Humalog® Novolin® NovoRapid®	2°C – 8°C 2°C – 10°C	3 weeks Use as quickly as possible

*Syringes should not be prepared in advance when using Lantus® because the insulin will become cloudy.
Advance preparation of Apidra® and Levemir® should also be avoided because of a lack of data regarding its stability.

4

What should insulin look like?

Insulin comes in either a clear solution that resembles water or a cloudy suspension that is milky in appearance.

CLEAR INSULIN		CLOUDY INSULIN	
Rapid:	• Apidra® • Humalog® • NovoRapid®	Intermediate:	• Humulin® N • Novolin® ge NPH
Fast:	• Humulin® R • Novolin® ge Toronto	Premixed:	• Humulin® 30/70 • Humalog® Mix 25 • Humalog® Mix 50 • Novolin® ge 30/70 • Novolin® ge 40/60 • Novolin® ge 50/50 • NovoMix® 30
Long:	• Lantus® • Levemir®		

When should clear insulin be discarded?

Clear insulin should be discarded if:

- it looks cloudy;
- it is thick;
- the solution contains solid particles;
- it has been exposed to extreme temperatures (heat or cold);
- the expiry date has passed.

What precautions should be taken with cloudy insulin?

Cloudy insulin is a suspension that needs to be mixed well before being used.

A whitish deposit at the bottom of the vial or in the cartridge is normal, but it must be remixed into the suspension. The vial should be rolled between the palms and turned upside down, or the cartridge should be turned over in the pen injector several times. **Do not shake.**

Improperly mixed cloudy insulin can make measured doses less precise.

When should cloudy insulin be discarded?

Cloudy insulin should be discarded if:

- a deposit remains at the bottom of the vial or in the cartridge;
- there are specks floating in the insulin;
- particles are stuck to the sides of the vial or cartridge, making the containers look frosted;
- it has been exposed to extreme temperatures (heat or cold);
- the expiry date has passed.

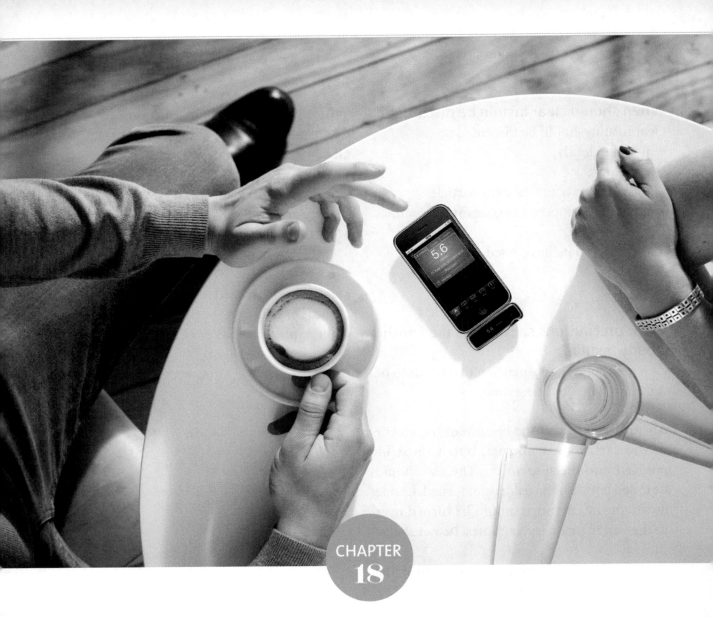

Insulin
Dose Adjustment

Why do insulin doses need to be adjusted?

The goal of insulin dose adjustment is to improve the control of blood glucose. Ideally, people with diabetes adjust their own doses after being shown how to do it by their health care team.

What are the target blood glucose levels when adjusting insulin doses?

Most people with diabetes should aim for blood glucose levels between 4 mmol/L and 7 mmol/L before meals and between 5 mmol/L and 10 mmol/L two hours after meals. A target blood glucose level between 5 mmol/L and 8 mmol/L two hours after a meal is possible if glycated hemoglobin (A1C) remains above 7%. A1C and blood glucose targets can be tailored to individuals on the basis of various factors (e.g., age, associated diseases, risk of severe hypoglycemia, etc.). The health care team should then explain these targets to the person with diabetes.

What are the rules governing insulin dose adjustment?

The rules in this section are a guide to making decisions about insulin dose adjustment and will ensure that any changes made are safe.

Here are the two basic principles:
- insulin lowers blood glucose levels;
- current blood glucose reflects what happened before.

Before adjusting an insulin dose, take the time to analyze blood glucose levels by calculating the average of the last three readings for each time of day (morning, noon, evening and bedtime), going back a maximum of seven days. Only levels recorded since the last adjustment should be considered.

The six rules for adjusting insulin doses are the following:

1 When calculating the average, do not take into account any measurement below 4 mmol/L or above 7 mmol/L that is associated with an isolated, exceptional or explainable situation.

2 Avoid adjusting insulin doses based on a single blood glucose test. Generally speaking, adjusting an insulin dose to correct blood glucose at one moment is not recommended.

3 Adjust one insulin dose at a time, for one time of day.

4 Correct **hypoglycemia** first, starting with the first of the day, then the second, and so on.

- **Hypoglycemia** can be identified by the following:
  - the average is below 4 mmol/L for a given period of the day;
  - the last two readings or three non-consecutive readings over the last seven days have revealed hypoglycemia, even if the average for a given time of day is greater than or equal to 4 mmol/L,
- A value of 2 mmol/L is assigned to any hypoglycemia that has not been measured.
- A hypoglycemic reading taken outside the four usual blood glucose measuring periods should be recorded under the following period (for example, a hypoglycemic reading measured in the morning should be recorded in the "before lunch" column).

5 Next, correct **hyperglycemic situations**, that is, situations in which average blood glucose at a given time of day is higher than 7 mmol/L. Begin with the first episode of the day, then the second, and so on.

Watch out for rebound hyperglycemia. Rebound hyperglycemia is a blood glucose reading above 7 mmol/L that follows hypoglycemia. This type of hyperglycemia should not be included when calculating the average. Nocturnal hypoglycemia can cause rebound hyperglycemia upon waking. When in doubt, take a blood glucose reading around 2 a.m. and if necessary correct the hypoglycemia instead of the morning hyperglycemia.

6 Wait at least two days after an adjustment before making any new modifications. The only exception is when there are two consecutive hypoglycemic readings. If that happens, disregard the rule and increase the dose of insulin that caused it.

What are the most frequently prescribed insulin regimens?

There are a number of different insulin regimens. The four most commonly prescribed are the following.

The basal-prandial regimen involves the injection of one rapid-acting (Apidra®, Humalog® or NovoRapid®) or short-acting insulin (Humulin® R or Novolin® ge Toronto) before each meal and one intermediate-acting (Humulin® N or Novolin® ge NPH) or long-acting insulin (Lantus® or Levemir®) at bedtime. Although basal insulin is usually administered in one injection, it can also be administered in more than one injection over the course of the day. The dose of rapid-acting or short-acting insulin can be fixed (fixed carbohydrate regimen) or based on the amount of carbohydrates consumed in a meal (variable carbohydrate regimen). Rapid-acting insulin is prescribed essentially for the variable carbohydrate regimen, in which the dose is expressed as a ratio such as 1 unit/10 g of carbohydrates (1 unit of insulin for every 10 g of carbohydrates consumed). Some people express this ratio in terms of grams of carbohydrates to units of insulin. In such a case, for example, the dose would be 15 g/1unit or 20 g/unit.

The **split-mixed regimen** involves injecting one intermediate-acting insulin (e.g. Humulin® N or Novolin® ge NPH) and one rapid-acting (Apidra®, Humalog® or NovoRapid®) or short-acting insulin (Humulin® R or Novolin® ge Toronto) before breakfast and dinner. Sometimes, the injection of intermediate-acting insulin before dinner needs to be delayed until bedtime to avoid nocturnal hypoglycemia.

The **premixed regimen** involves injecting one premixed insulin (for example, Humulin® 30/70, Novolin® ge 50/50, Humalog®Mix 25, NovoMix®30, etc.) before breakfast and dinner.

The **combined regimen** involves injecting one intermediate-acting insulin (Humulin® N or Novolin® ge NPH) or long-acting insulin (Lantus® and Levemir®) at bedtime in combination with antidiabetic drugs during the day.

In the basal-prandial regimen, which insulins affect blood glucose levels measured during the day?

The type of insulin	is responsible	for the blood glucose measured:
Intermediate- or long-acting at bedtime	⟶	before breakfast
Rapid- or short-acting at breakfast	⟶	before lunch
Rapid- or short-acting at lunchtime	⟶	before dinner
Rapid- or short-acting at dinner	⟶	at bedtime (before snack)

Blood glucose levels at any given moment always reflect the action of the insulin injected before.

How should insulin doses be adjusted in the basal-prandial with fixed carbohydrates regimen?

In general, when **hypoglycemia (average blood glucose below 4 mmol/L)** occurs before meals and at bedtime (as defined in the adjustment rules), the insulin dose should be decreased by 2 units at a time. However, if the total **daily dose** of insulin is less than or equal to 20 units, the dose that caused it should be reduced by one unit at a time.

In general, when **hyperglycemia (average blood glucose above 7 mmol/L)** occurs before meals and at bedtime (as defined in the adjustment rules), the insulin dose should be **increased** by two units at a time. However, if the total **daily dose** of insulin is less than or equal to 20 units, the dose that caused it should be increased by one unit at a time.

Wait at least two days after any insulin dose adjustment before making any new changes. The only exception is in the event of two consecutive episodes of hypoglycemia in the same period. In such a case, disregard the rule and decrease the dose of insulin that caused it. In the event of hypoglycemia or hyperglycemia, never wait more than one week before adjusting the dose that caused it.

How should insulin doses be adjusted in the basal-prandial with variable carbohydrate regimen?

When **hypoglycemia (average blood glucose below 4 mmol/L)** occurs, as defined in the adjustment rules:

- overnight or before breakfast, the inter-mediate-acting insulin (e.g. Humulin® or Novolin® ge NPH) or long-acting insulin (Lantus® or Levemir®) should be **decreased** by 2 units at a time. However, if the daily intermediate- or long-acting insulin dose is less than or equal to 10 units, the dose should be decreased by only 1 unit at a time;
- before lunch, dinner, or bedtime, the insulin dose responsible (e.g., Apidra®, Humalog®, or NovoRapid®) should be **decreased** by 0.2 units/10 g of carbohydrates at a time. However, if this insulin dose was less than or equal to 0.5 units/10 g of carbohydrates, the dose should be decreased by only 0.1 unit/10 g of carbohydrates at a time.

When **hyperglycemia (average blood glucose above 7 mmol/L)** occurs, as defined in the adjustment rules:

- overnight or before breakfast, the intermediate-acting insulin (e.g. Humulin® or Novolin® ge NPH) or long-acting insulin (Lantus® or Levemir®) should be **increased** by 2 units at a time. However, if the daily dose of intermediate- or long-acting insulin is less than or equal to 10 units, the dose should be increased by only one unit at a time.
- before lunch, dinner, or bedtime, the insulin dose responsible (e.g., Apidra®, Humalog®, or NovoRapid®) should be **increased** by 0.2 units/10 g of carbohydrates at a time. However, if this insulin dose was less than or equal to 0.5 units/10 g of carbohydrates, the dose should be increased by only 0.1 unit/10 g of carbohydrates at a time.

Wait at least two days after any insulin dose adjustment before making any new changes. The only exception is in the event of two consecutive episodes of hypoglycemia in the same period. In such a case, disregard the rule and decrease the dose of insulin that caused it. In the event of hypoglycemia or hyperglycemia, never wait longer than one week before adjusting the dose that caused it.

In the split-mixed regimen, which insulins affect blood glucose levels during the day?

The type of insulin	is responsible	for the blood glucose measured:
Intermediate-acting before dinner	⟶	before breakfast
Rapid-or short-acting before breakfast	⟶	before lunch
Intermediate-acting at breakfast	⟶	before dinner
Rapid-or short-acting before dinner	⟶	At bedtime (before snack)

Blood glucose levels at any given moment reflect the action of the insulin injected before.

9

How should insulin doses be adjusted in the split-mixed regimen?

In general, when **hypoglycemia (average blood glucose below 4 mmol/L)** as defined in the adjustment rules occurs before meals and at bedtime, the insulin dose should be **decreased** by 2 units at a time. However, if the **total daily dose** of insulin is less than or equal to 20 units, the dose that caused it should be reduced by only 1 unit at a time.

In general, when **hyperglycemia (average blood glucose above 7 mmol/L)** as defined in the adjustment rules occurs before meals and at bedtime, the insulin dose should be **increased** by 2 units at a time. However, if the **total daily dose** of insulin is less than or equal to 20 units, the dose that caused it should be increased by only one unit at a time.

Wait at least two days after any insulin dose adjustment before making any new changes. The only exception is in the event of two consecutive episodes of hypoglycemia in the same period. In such a case, disregard the rule and decrease the dose of insulin that caused it. In the event of hypoglycemia or hyperglycemia, never wait more than one week before adjusting the dose that caused it.

10

In the premixed regimen, which insulins affect blood glucose levels at different times of day?

The type of insulin	affects	the blood glucose measured:
Rapid- or short-acting and intermediate-acting in the morning		before lunch and before dinner
Rapid- or short-acting and intermediate-acting at dinner		At bedtime (before snack) and before breakfast

Blood glucose levels at any given moment reflect the action of the insulin injected before.

11

How should insulin doses be adjusted in the premixed regimen?

In general, when **hypoglycemia (average blood glucose below 4 mmol/L)** as defined in the adjustment rules occurs before meals and at bedtime, the mixed insulin dose that caused it should be **decreased** by 2 units at a time. However, if the **total daily dose** of insulin is less than or equal to 20 units, the dose should be reduced by only one unit at a time.

In general, when hyperglycemia (average blood glucose above 7mmol/L) as defined in the adjustment rules occurs, the mixed insulin dose that caused it should be increased by two units at a time. However, if the total daily dose of insulin is less than or equal to 20 units, the dose should be increased by only one unit at a time.

Remember that premixed insulins are responsible for two periods of the day at a time. Therefore, if there is a difference between the blood glucose at bedtime and that in the morning (for example, high at bedtime and low in the morning) or between the blood glucose before lunch and that before dinner, you should see a doctor because this could mean that the mixture needs to be changed.

Wait at least two days after any insulin dose adjustment before making any new changes. The only exception is in the event of two consecutive episodes of hypoglycemia in the same period. In such a case, disregard the rule and decrease the dose of insulin that caused it. In the event of hypoglycemia or hyperglycemia, never wait more than one week before adjusting the dose that caused it.

In the combined regimen, which blood glucose reading is affected by insulin administered at bedtime?

In the combined regimen, morning blood glucose is affected by the intermediate-acting or long-acting insulin administered at bedtime.

How should insulin doses be adjusted in the combined regimen?

In general, when morning hypoglycemia (average blood glucose below 4mmol/L) as defined in the adjustment rules occurs, the bedtime insulin dose should be decreased by two units at a time. However, if the total daily dose of insulin is less than or equal to 10 units, the dose should be reduced by only one unit.

In general, when morning hyperglycemia (average blood glucose above 7mmol/L) as defined in the adjustment rules occurs, the bedtime insulin dose should be increased by two units at a time. However, if the total daily dose of insulin is less than or equal to 10 units, the dose should be increased by only one unit.

Wait at least two days after any insulin dose adjustment before making any new changes. The only exception is in the event of two consecutive episodes of hypoglycemia in the same period. In such a case, disregard the rule and decrease the dose of insulin that caused it. In the event of hypoglycemia or hyperglycemia, never wait more than one week before adjusting the dose that caused.

Are there different ways of adjusting insulin doses?

Different methods can be applied when adjusting insulin doses. Sometimes, especially in the basal-prandial regimen, the method involves corrective doses, which are established by the health care team on the basis of the total daily insulin dose and what is referred to as the insulin sensitivity factor. Corrective doses are supplements of rapid-acting insulin or, less frequently, short-acting insulin (the same type used at meals) taken in addition to the meal dose if blood glucose is higher than a determined value. Corrective doses can be useful in some circumstances, particularly when the person with diabetes is ill and blood glucose is higher.

An adjustment based on the tendency of blood glucose levels, as described in the rules of adjustment, is to be preferred. Corrective doses are not an essential component of insulin therapy and can sometimes be overused, leading to significant fluctuations in blood glucose. If one period of the day requires several corrective doses over a single week (e.g., correction required at breakfast because of high blood glucose in the morning), the dose of insulin that caused it needs to be readjusted – in other words, the long-acting insulin taken at bedtime, responsible for the morning blood glucose, should be increased. For more details, see the chapter on pump therapy.

Take-home message: The self-adjustment of insulin doses requires appropriate instructions from the health care team.

PRACTICAL EXAMPLES

It is important to understand the rules of adjustment described in this chapter before attempting any insulin dose adjustment. The following practical examples can be useful:

Example 1:

TREATMENT: BASAL-PRANDIAL WITH FIXED CARBOHYDRATES REGIMEN

NovoRapid®
• 8 units at breakfast, 6 units at lunch, 6 units at dinner

Novolin® ge NPH:
• 16 units at bedtime

Total daily insulin dose = 36 units

Self-monitoring logbook

Date	BLOOD GLUCOSE			
	Before breakfast (mmol/L)	Before lunch (mmol/L)	Before dinner (mmol/L)	At bedtime (mmol/L)
03/01	12	9	8	6.5
04/01	13	8.7	7.2	5.8
05/01	11.7	8.9	7.8	5.6
Average	12.2	8.9	7.7	6.0

Analysis

In this example, hyperglycemia occurs before breakfast, lunch and dinner. The first period of hyperglycemia to be corrected should be the first one of the day, which occurred before breakfast. The insulin to adjust is the bedtime NPH, which should be increased by 2 units to 18 units. However, blood glucose should be checked at 2 a.m. to rule out nocturnal hypoglycemia that could cause a rebound hyperglycemia in the morning. If hypoglycemia does occur during the night, the NPH insulin at bedtime should be decreased by 2 units.

Example 2
TREATMENT: BASAL-PRANDIAL WITH VARIABLE CARBOHYDRATE REGIMEN

Apidra®

1.2 units/10 g of carbohydrates at breakfast
1.0 units/10 g of carbohydrates at lunch
0.8 units/10 g of carbohydrates at dinner

Lantus®

12 units at bedtime

Self-monitoring logbook

| Date | BLOOD GLUCOSE | | | |
	Before breakfast (mmol/L)	Before lunch (mmol/L)	Before dinner (mmol/L)	At bedtime (mmol/L)
13/04	5.4	6.4	4.4	5.8
14/04	5.9	6.0	3.6	5.0
15/04	5.3	5.6	2.8	5.2
Average	5.5	6.0	3.6	5.3

Analysis

In this example, two episodes of **hypoglycemia** are measured in the two blood glucose readings taken before dinner. The appropriate adjustment would be to **decrease** the insulin at dinner by 0.2 units/10 g of carbohydrates, from 1.0 units/10 g to 0.8 units/10 g of carbohydrates.

Example 3
TREATMENT: SPLIT-MIXED REGIMEN

Humulin® R
· 12 units at breakfast and 10 units at dinner

Humulin® N
· 20 units at breakfast and 14 units at dinner

Total daily insulin dose = 56 units

Self-monitoring logbook

Date	BLOOD GLUCOSE			
	Before breakfast (mmol/L)	Before lunch (mmol/L)	Before dinner (mmol/L)	At bedtime (mmol/L)
16/05	6.4	7.7	6.5	5.7
17/05	7.1	9.3	7.0	5.4
18/05	5.9	7.5	6.2	6.0
Average	6.5	8.2	6.6	5.7

Analysis

In this example, the average blood glucose before lunch is higher than 7 mmol/L (hyperglycemia). The appropriate adjustment would be to increase the morning dose of rapid-acting insulin by 2 units. The breakfast dose of Humulin®R should therefore be increased to 14 units.

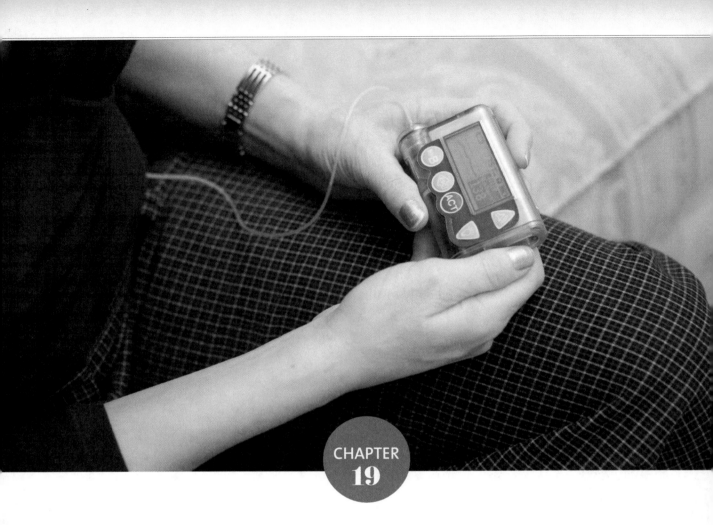

CHAPTER
19

The Insulin Pump:
Another Treatment Option[1]

What is an insulin pump?

An insulin pump is a device consisting of:
- a reservoir or cartridge containing insulin;
- an electric motor to deliver insulin from the reservoir;
- a cannula, or small tube, attached to the insulin reservoir and fitted with a small needle that is inserted beneath the skin of the abdomen, where the insulin is injected.

The OmniPod® is a new insulin-delivery system that has recently become available. The Pod is a self-adhesive device containing an insulin reservoir, a motor, and a small, flexible tube through which the insulin is delivered. This system does not include a cannula. A wireless device is used to program the Pod remotely and contains an integrated blood glucose meter.

An insulin pump administers insulin subcutaneously on a continual basis, 24 hours a day; this is the basal rate. The **basal rate** fills insulin needs without taking meals into consideration. The pump can be programmed to provide different basal rates to meet insulin needs that vary according to the time of day. Before meals, an extra dose is injected via the pump to provide insulin required for meals; this is the bolus dose. The continual release of insulin along with the pre-meal bolus imitates the normal function of the pancreas. Generally, insulin pumps use rapid-acting insulin such as Apidra®, Humalog® or NovoRapid®. The insulin pump is not an artificial pancreas. It does only what it is programmed to do.

What are the indications for using an insulin pump?

Current indications for using an insulin pump tend to be restrictive because the equipment is expensive. The following indications are usually recognized:
- serious hypoglycemia (requiring the help of a third person) on more than one occasion;
- high glucose lability (instability) requiring repeated medical attention on more than one occasion;
- inadequate control of blood glucose despite an attempt at intensive insulin therapy;
- accelerated progression of complications (retinopathy and/or neuropathy) with suboptimal blood glucose control (glycosylated hemoglobin > 7%).

The insulin pump can also be an option for the following individuals:
- a pregnant woman;
- a diabetic person who wants to intensify treatment;
- a person with a very irregular schedule or very active lifestyle.

1 Canadian Diabetes Association Clinical Practice Guidelines Expert Committee. Canadian Diabetes Association 2013 Clinical Practice Guidelines for the Prevention and Management of Diabetes in Canada. *Can. J. Diabetes* 2013; 37(suppl 1):S1-S212.

How much does insulin pump treatment cost?

An insulin pump costs approximately $6,500, and the material required (needles, catheters, insulin, etc.) can cost between $2,000 and $4,000 a year.

Is insulin pump treatment covered by medical insurance?

Since 2011, the Quebec drug insurance plan has covered the cost of the purchase of an insulin pump and the material required for children under the age of 18 with type 1 diabetes, and continues paying for them after they become adults. It does not cover these costs if an individual begins using the pump as an adult, however. Some private insurance companies cover up to 80% of the costs, provided they accept the justification for this type of treatment. Other companies contribute a maximum, non-renewable amount.

In Ontario, the pump is covered for children and eligible adults with type 1 diabetes.

What should I do if I think I could benefit from insulin pump treatment?

First, discuss it with your endocrinologist. If insulin pump treatment is appropriate:

1 check with your insurance company to see whether it covers insulin pump treatment;
2 ask your doctor for the following:
   - a prescription for the pump;
   - a letter attesting that insulin pump treatment is indicated, to be submitted to your insurance company.

What are the procedures for using an insulin pump?

A qualified health care team must provide instructions on how to use an insulin pump, and an endocrinologist prescribes and adjusts insulin doses. The instructions the individual receives should include a description of:

- how the pump functions;
- how to install the cannula and how to choose the injection area; and
- how to calculate carbohydrates;
- how to self-adjust insulin doses.

Ask your endocrinologist about the procedures to follow and the people to contact.

How is the dosage determined for insulin pumps?

Generally, rapid-acting insulin (Apidra®, Humalog® or NovoRapid®) is used. To determine the basal dose, begin with 50% of the total insulin dose for the day in your prior treatment (e.g., if your total dose of rapid- and long-acting insulin for 24 hours was 40 units, the basal dose with the pump should be 40 ÷ 2 = 20 units).

When determining the daily distribution of the basal dose, take the following two factors into account: 1) generally speaking, people are most sensitive to insulin between midnight and 4 a.m. and are therefore the most vulnerable to hypoglycemia during these hours, and 2) people are generally most resistant to insulin between 4 a.m. to 8 a.m and therefore need more insulin during this period. Therefore, the midnight basal rate should be decreased by 25% and the 4 a.m. rate increased by 25% to 50%.

For example, if the amount of insulin is 20 units every 24 hours, the basal rate is 0.8 units/hour (20 units ÷ 24 hours = 0.8 units/hour). However, taking the information above into account, the basal rate should be lowered by 25% between midnight and 4 a.m. (to 0.6 units/hour) and increased by 50% between 4 a.m. and 8 a.m. (to 1.2 units/hour).

There are different methods to calculate the **pre-meal bolus** dose:

- begin with 1.0 unit per 10 g of carbohydrates for each meal, then adjust the dose as needed. For example, a meal containing 60 g of carbohydrates requires a dose of 6 units: (60 g ÷ 10 g) x 1.0 unit = 6 units.
- Apply the "**Rule of 500**": divide 500 by the total daily insulin dose (to be administered over 24 hours). For example, if your total daily dose is 40 units, 1.0 unit of insulin should be administered for every 12 g of carbohydrates: 500 ÷ 40 = 12.5.
- Use the insulin ratios from your prior multiple injection treatment as a guide.

Are there always different basal rates for different times of day?

Not necessarily. However, there are five distinct periods in a day, and basal requirements can vary with each one

Period 1: 12 a.m. (midnight) to 4 a.m. People are most vulnerable to hypoglycemia during these hours and it may be necessary to deliver less insulin.

Period 2: 4 a.m. to 8 a.m. People are more insulin-resistant during this period and may need more insulin.

Period 3: 8 a.m. to 12 p.m. (noon). This is a more active period of the day and may require a lower basal rate.

Period 4: 12 p.m. (noon) to 6 p.m. This is a more active period of the day and may require a lower basal rate.

Period 5: 6 p.m. to 12 a.m. (midnight). This less active period may require a higher basal rate.

These periods may vary in terms of their precise times depending on the individual's lifestyle.

Which blood glucose readings are used to adjust the basal rate for each period?

It is important to identify the blood glucose readings during the day that reflect the basal rate for each period. These readings can be used as a basis for making adjustments.

Period		Basal blood glucose
Midnight to 4 a.m.	⟶	Around 3 a.m or 4 a.m.
4 a.m. to 8 a.m.	⟶	Before breakfast (around 7 a.m. or 8 a.m.
8 a.m. to noon	⟶	Before lunch (around 11 a.m. or noon)
Noon to 6 p.m.	⟶	Before dinner (between 4 p.m. and 6 p.m.)
6 p.m. to midnight	⟶	At bedtime (around 11 p.m. or midnight)

Which blood glucose readings are used to adjust the pre-meal bolus dose?

The bolus for each meal is adjusted according to the postprandial blood glucose reading (2 hours after the beginning of the meal).

Meal		Postprandial blood glucose (2 hours after meal)
Breakfast	⟶	After breakfast
Lunch	⟶	After lunch
Dinner	⟶	After dinner

What are the target blood glucose levels?

Basal blood glucose: Most people are advised to target a blood glucose level between 4 mmol/L and 7 mmol/L before meals and at bedtime (before the snack).

Postprandial blood glucose: The recommended postprandial blood glucose level is higher than the pre-meal blood glucose. In most cases, target postprandial blood glucose should be between 5 mmol/L and 10 mmol/L (2 hours after the beginning of the meal). After-meal targets should be tailored to individuals. If diabetes control is not optimal (glycated hemoglobin greater than 7%), the target should be between 5 mmol/L and 8 mmol/L.

What are the insulin adjustment rules?

Before adjusting your insulin doses, take the time to analyze your blood glucose by calculating the average of the last two or three readings for each period of the day (before meals, after meals, and bedtime), going back no further than seven days. Only readings done since the last adjustment should be taken into account.

Here are a few rules to guide adjustment:

1 When calculating the average, do not take into account any measurements lower than 4 mmol/L or higher than 7mmol/L that are associated with an **isolated, exceptional and explainable situation.**

2 Avoid adjusting insulin doses based on only **one blood glucose reading**. Adjusting insulin dosage to correct blood glucose at any one given moment is generally discouraged.

3 Adjust **only one insulin dose** at a time (basal rate or bolus) and for one period of the day only.

4 Adjust the basal rate before re-evaluating the bolus.

5 Correct hypoglycemia first, starting with the first of the day.
- **Basal hypoglycemia** occurs when:
  - the basal blood glucose average for a given period of the day is below 4 mmol/L;
  - the last two readings for the same time of day indicate hypoglycemia or, over the last seven days, three non-consecutive readings for the same time of day indicate hypoglycemia, even if the average is equal to or greater than 4 mmol/L.
- **Postprandial hypoglycemia** occurs when:
  - average postprandial blood glucose levels after a given meal are lower than average blood glucose levels before the same meal;
  - the last two postprandial readings reveal blood glucose levels lower than before the meal or, over the last seven days, three non-consecutive postprandial readings reveal blood glucose lower than before the meal, even if the average postprandial levels are higher than the average levels before the meal.
- Assign a value of 2 mmol/L to any hypoglycemia that has not been measured.
- Hypoglycemia that occurs outside the usual blood glucose measuring periods should be recorded under the following period (for example, hypoglycemia at 11 a.m. is entered in the "before lunch" column).

6 Next, correct **hyperglycemia**, which occurs when the basal blood glucose level for the same time of day is greater than 7 mmol/L or the postprandial blood glucose level is greater than 10 mmol/L. Begin with the first of the day, then the second, and so on.
Watch out for rebound hyperglycemia. Rebound hyperglycemia is a basal blood glucose level above 7mmol/L that follows hypoglycemia. This type of hyperglycemia should not be included when calculating the average.

7 If possible, wait at least two days after adjusting a dose before making any other changes.

How should insulin doses be adjusted?

The methods for adjusting subcutaneous insulin pump therapy will not be discussed in detail, as instruction from a specialized team is required. A useful reference book, however, is *Pumping Insulin*, by John Walsh and Ruth Roberts.

This section will outline a few basic concepts regarding the rules of adjustment.

The basal rate is determined according to blood glucose measured at 3 a.m. or 4 a.m., before meals, and at bedtime. The bolus rate is determined according to blood glucose measured 2 hours after the beginning of a meal. These values are used to adjust insulin doses as follows:

Basal rate:

- If hypoglycemic, decrease the corresponding basal rate by 0.1 unit/hour to 0.2 units/hour.
- If hyperglycemic, increase the corresponding basal rate by 0.1 unit/hour to 0.2 units/hour.

Bolus:

- If hypoglycemic, increase the amount of carbohydrates per unit of insulin (e.g., if the current bolus is 1.0 unit of insulin per 12 g of carbohydrates, change it to 1.0 unit of insulin per 13 g of carbohydrates). If the dose is expressed in units of insulin per 10 g of carbohydrates, decrease the number of units

per 10 g (e.g., from 1.0 unit/10 g to 0.8 unit/10 g).

- If hyperglycemic, decrease the number of carbohydrates per unit of insulin (e.g., if the current bolus is 1.0 unit of insulin per 12 g of carbohydrates, change it to 1.0 unit of insulin per 11 g of carbohydrates). If the dose is expressed in units of insulin per 10 g of carbohydrates, increase the number of units per 10 g (e.g., from 1.0 unit/10 g to 1.2 unit/10 g).

What is a correction dose and a sensitivity factor?

If your blood glucose is higher or lower than the target you set with your endocrinologist, you should increase or decrease the amount of insulin planned for the bolus dose. This is a correction dose.

To determine the proper correction dose, you have to determine your insulin sensitivity factor. Your sensitivity factor indicates the expected decrease in blood glucose when you take 1 unit of insulin. It is calculated by dividing 100 by the daily total insulin dose (over 24 hours). For example, if your total daily dose is 40 units, your sensitivity factor is $100 \div 40 = 2.5$. Thus, 1 unit of insulin decreases blood glucose by about 2.5 mmol/L.

To calculate the correction dose by which your regular bolus dose should be increased or decreased, subtract your target blood glucose level from your current blood glucose level and divide it by your sensitivity factor. Here are two examples:

1 **Blood glucose higher than the target:**
   Current blood glucose level = 11 mmol/L
   Target blood glucose level = 5.5 mmol/L
   Sensitivity factor = 2.5.
   Correction dose = (11 - 5.5) ÷ 2.5 = 2.2
   Therefore, you should add 2.2 units of insulin to your regular bolus dose.

2 **Blood glucose lower than the target:**
   Current blood glucose level: 3.5 mmol/L
   Target blood glucose level: 5.5 mmol/L
   Sensitivity factor: 2.5
   Correction dose = (3.5 - 5.5) ÷ 2.5 = - 0.8.
   Therefore, you should subtract 0.8 units of insulin from your regular bolus dose.

Calculation of insulin sensitivity factor (ISF):
Rule of 100
ISF = 100 ÷ TDD = X

⬇

1 unit of insulin decreases blood glucose by X mmol/L

(TDD: total daily dose of insulin)

Calculation of correction dose:
Correction dose =
(current blood glucose - target blood glucose) ÷ ISF

If current blood glucose is higher than the target, the correction dose will be a positive value.

If current blood glucose is lower than the target, the correction dose will be a negative value.

If several correction doses are necessary for the same period in the same week (e.g., corrections needed at breakfast because blood glucose is high in the morning), the insulin dose that caused it must be adjusted (e.g., increase the basal flow for the second part of the night, after 4 a.m., which is responsible for morning blood glucose levels).

When should the injection site be changed?

Immediately:
- if you feel pain or discomfort;
- if two correction bolus doses do not reduce high blood glucose (blocked cannula);
- if there are ketone bodies in your blood or urine with no explanation;
- if you observe blood in the cannula.

Every 24 to 48 hours:
- if you use a steel needle set;
- if you are pregnant.

Every 48 to 72 hours:
- if you use a soft cannula set.

In general, it is recommended to **replace the perfusion device – that is, the reservoir, the tubing, the cannula or the Pod — every 48 to 72 hours.** The suggested frequency varies depending on the type of pump, the brand of insulin, and the choice of cannula.

Be careful of any failure of the pump or any problem with the cannula. Ketoacidosis can develop more quickly and more frequently when using the pump instead of the basal-prandial regimen because your body lacks insulin reserves. Always have a pen device with rapid-acting and long-acting insulin on hand. If your blood glucose rises above 14 mmol/l, take a ketone body reading (see Chapter 21). If you detect ketone bodies or if hyperglycemia persists, take your correction dose with the pen device and call your doctor or go to the emergency room.

What types of insulin pumps are available in Canada?

The following table presents a list of the latest generation of insulin pumps on the market, as well as a few of their features. This list was revised on May 1, 2013, and was adapted from a document entitled *"Comparaison des pompes à insuline"* from the Centre hospitalier universitaire de Québec (Quebec University Hospital).

Model	Manufacturer or distributor	Weight of pump (grams)	
ACCU-CHEK®V SPIRIT COMBO	Roche Diagnostics Canada	110	
ANIMAS® ONE TOUCH PING	Johnson & Johnson	110	
MINIMED® PARADIGM® VEO®	Medtronic		
VEO 554		100	
VEO 754		108	
OMNIPOD®	Glaxo SmithKline Inc.	Pod: 34 PDM: 125 (personal diabetes manager)	

Size (cm)	Colour	Screen	Reservoir (units)	Connection	Battery lifespan (weeks)	Water-tightness
8.3 x 5.6 x 2.1	black	Colour LCD with backlilght	315	Luer lock	If Bluetooth® is activated, 11 (lithium AA x 1) 4 (alkaline AA x 1) 5 to 6 (NiMH HR6 AA rechargeable	60 mins at 2.5 metres
5.1 x 7.7 x 1.8	5 colours (black, blue, green, pink, grey)	Colour LED, high contrast with backlight	200	Luer lock	6 to 8 lithium AA x 1) 2 to 3 (alkaline AA x 1)	24 hrs at 3.6 metres
8.3 X 5.0 X 2.0 9.5 X 5.0 X 2.0	Clear, blue, smoked, purple, pink	With backlight	176 300	Paradigm exclusive	2 to 4 (alkaline AAA x 1)	Water resistant
Pod: 4.1 X 6.2 X 1.7 GPD: 6.4 X 11.4 X 2.5	Pod: white PDM: blu	LCD	200	Pod without cannula	3 (alkaline AAA x 2)	Pod: 60 mins at 706 metres PDM: not watertight

Model	Basal delivery (min/max) in units/hour	Increase in basal flow units/hour	Basal release	Temporary basal rate	Bolus (min/max) in units	Length of bolus for 1 unit	
ACCU-CHEK®V SPIRIT COMBO	0.05 to 5.0	0.01 (up to 1) 0.05 (up to 10) 0.1 (up to 50)	Every 3 mins	0% to 250% 15 mins to 24 hrs	0.1 to 50 units (in increments of 0.1, 0.2, 0.5, 1.0 and 2.0)	5 secs	
ANIMAS® ONE TOUCH PING	0.025 to 25	0.025	Every 3 mins	-OFF -90% to 200% 30 mins to 24 hours	0.05 to 35 units (increments of 0.05)	1 or 4 secs	
MINIMED® PARADIGM® VEO® VEO 554 VEO 754	0.025 to 35	0.025	Total dose administerd over 60 mins in increments of 0.05 (or increments of 0.025 when total hourly dose is less than 1 unit)	0% to 200% 30 mins to 24 hrs	0.025 to 75 units (increments of 0.025 – 0.05 – 0.1)	40 secs	
OMNIPOD®	0.05 to 30	0.05	Total dose administered over 60 minutes in increments of 0.05	-100% to 95% 30 mins to 12 hours	0.05 to 30 (increments of 0.05 - 0.01 - 0.50 - 1.0	40 secs	

Download software	Blood glucose meter	Specific features	Price	Technical support and internet address
Accu-check® 360 version 2.0	Accu-Chek® Aviva Combo	Meter also remotely controls the pump. Blood glucose meter with colour screen. Reversible pump screen (180 degrees)	$6,395	1-800-688-4578 www.accu-chek.ca
Diasend® (web-based) or ez-Manager Max® (PC or Mac)	One Touch® Ping®	Blood glucose meter with integrated remote. Possibility to record carbohydrate content of 500 foods. Pump 100% watertight	$6,895 for Ping® system (pump and meter)	1-866-406-4844 www.animas.ca
CareLink™ Personal (carelink. minimed.com)	Contour® Link	Continuous blood glucose monitoring integrated into pump (option). Graphic display of last 3, 6, 12 or 24 hours. Alarms (hypo-hyper, and suspension for hypoglycemia with option for continuous blood glucose). New Enlite® sensor (can be worn for 6 days)	$7,000 (MiniLink™ transmitter 799$ including box of 5 Enlite sensors)	1-800-284-4416 www.medtronic diabete.ca
FreeStyle® CoPilot health management system with OmniPod extension	FreeStyle® blood glucose meter integrated in the PDM (Personal Diabetes Manager)	Tubeless and waterproof Pod, automatic system to start Pod and injection process	$6,300 for PDM, $30 for Pod	1-855-763-4636 www.myomnipod.ca www.monomnipod.ca

1 Canadian Diabetes Association Clinical Practice Guidelines Expert Committee. Canadian Diabetes Association 2013 Clinical Practice Guidelines for the Prevention and Management of Diabetes in Canada. *Can. J. Diabetes* 2013; 37(suppl 1):S1-S212.

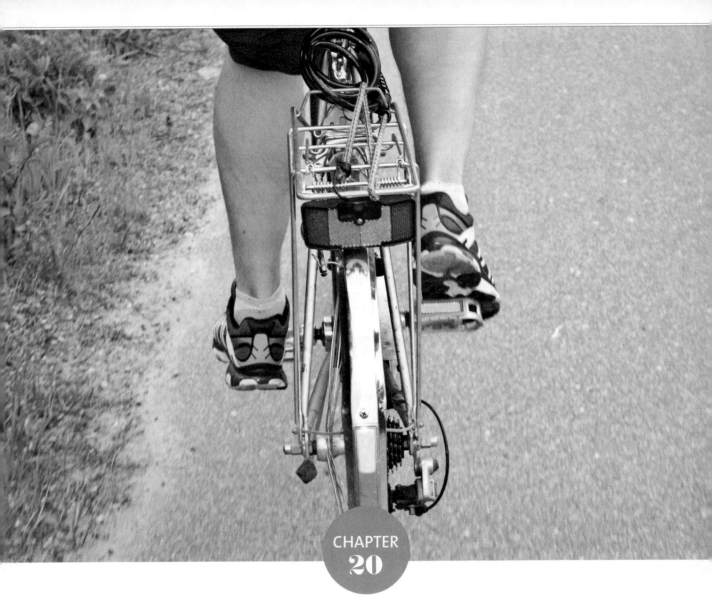

CHAPTER
20

Physical Activity

What is physical activity?

Physical activity is defined as any bodily movement produced by the muscles and requiring an additional expenditure of energy. There are two categories: aerobic physical activity and resistance physical activity. Aerobic physical activity involves the continuous movement of large muscle groups (for example, walking, cycling, running) for at least 10 consecutive minutes. Resistance physical activity is characterized by repetitions of brief exercises with free weights, machines, elastic bands, or one's own body weight (e.g., push-ups).

What are the risks of a lack of physical activity?

- Premature death;
- Heart disease;
- Obesity;
- High blood pressure;
- Diabetes;
- Osteoporosis;
- Stroke;
- Depression;
- Colon cancer.

What are the benefits of physical activity?

Regular exercise is beneficial for everyone, whether or not they have diabetes. Benefits include:

- Better health, improved physical fitness, increased self-esteem;
- Better posture and balance;
- Strengthening of the muscles and bones;
- Increased energy;
- Weight control;
- Lower blood lipid levels;
- Lower blood pressure;
- Relaxation and stress control;
- Increased autonomy in later years.

The benefits of aerobic activity:

Regular aerobic activity is associated with a decrease in mortality due to cardiovascular disease in people with either type 1 or type 2 diabetes. It is also associated with a slowing of the development of neuropathy and better glycemic control in people with type 2 diabetes.

The benefits of resistance activity:

Resistance activity is accompanied by lowered glycated hemoglobin (A1C), lowered insulin resistance, increased strength and muscle mass, and increased bone density.

What are the benefits of regular exercise for people with glucose intolerance (prediabetic state) or people with diabetes?

All types of activity are beneficial. People with glucose intolerance and people with diabetes derive the same benefits from exercise as people with normal glucose tolerance.

However, glucose-intolerant individuals who engage in regular, moderate physical activity reduce their risk of developing diabetes.

People with type 2 diabetes who engage in regular physical activity decrease their resistance to insulin and are better able to control their diabetes.

Regular exercise is also beneficial for people with type 1 diabetes. It is vital, however, that people with type 1 diabetes control the disease well and adapt their insulin doses and diet to their physical activity to prevent hypoglycemia or hyperglycemia.

How should a successful exercise program be approached?

First, choose a sport or activity that you like. Dancing, light gymnastics, swimming, working out at the gym, and brisk walking are all examples of simple and pleasant physical activities. The important thing is to choose something that appeals to you so that you will be more likely to do it on a daily basis.

Include the activity in your daily schedule.

Daily life offers a number of opportunities for exercise. For example, you can:
- walk or bike to work;
- take the stairs instead of the elevator;
- do manual tasks such as sweeping, cleaning windows, gardening, etc.

Is there an exercise program recommended to help control diabetes?

According to recent recommendations, all adults between 18 and 65 years old should engage in at least 150 minutes of moderate physical activity per week.

This activity should be spread over at least three days of the week, with no more than two consecutive days of inactivity. Possible schedules include:

- 50 minutes, 3 times a week (Mondays, Wednesdays and Saturdays, for example)
- or 30 minutes, 5 times a week
- Two or three exercise sessions a week should include resistance activities.

In one day, physical activity can be performed for the full 50 or 30 minutes consecutively or over several periods of at least 10 minutes each.

The most accessible exercise is brisk walking. Walking briskly, but still at a pace that allows conversation without breathlessness, is considered to be moderate exercise.

The energy expended by engaging in regular physical activity helps people maintain a healthy weight.

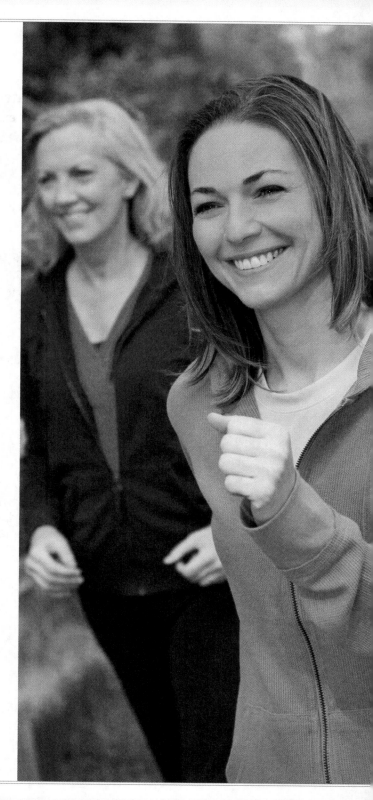

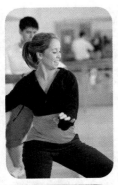

What are some low, moderate, and high intensity exercises?

The following chart ranks examples of physical activities according to the length and intensity of effort they require.

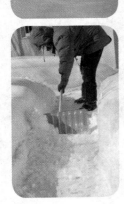

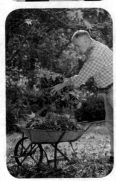

**LESS INTENSE
LONGER**

- Washing and waxing a car (45-60 mins)

- Washing floors and windows (45-60 mins)

- Gardening (30-45 mins)

- Moving around in a wheelchair (30-40 mins)

- Walking 3 km in 35 minutes (12 mins/km)

- Dancing (fast, for 30 mins)

- Walking with a baby (2.5 km in 30 mins)

- Raking leaves (30 mins)

- Walking 3.5 km in 30 minutes (8½ mins/km)

- Aquafitness (30 mins)

- Swimming (20 mins)

- Biking 6.5 km in 15 minutes

- Running 2.5 km in 15 minutes (6 mins/km)

- Shoveling snow or climbing stairs (15 mins)

**MORE INTENSE
SHORTER**

How do I ensure that my exercise is sufficiently intense but also pleasant and safe? How do I make sure that I progress at my own speed?

It is strongly recommended that people beginning an exercise program start out slowly and increase their pace little by little. Knowing how to pace yourself to be able to assess and develop your capacity for physical effort is critical. There are a number of ways to set your own pace.

Degree of breathlessness: Find the level where your breathing is deeper than when you are at rest but you are still able to have a conversation.

Pulse or heart rate (HR): Exercise is considered moderate when your pulse is between 50% and 70% of your maximum heart rate as assessed by a health professional (direct measurement). The following chart can help you determine whether the intensity of your exercise is appropriate

TIME NEEDED DEPENDS ON EFFORT

Very Light Effort	Light Effort 60 minutes	Moderate Effort 30-60 minutes	Vigorous Effort 20-30 minutes	Maximum Effort
• Strolling • Dusting	• Light walking • Volleyball • Easy gardening • Stretching	• Brisk walking • Biking • Raking leaves • Swimming • Dancing • Water aerobics	• Aerobics • Jogging • Hockey • Basketball • Fast swimming • Fast aerobics	• Sprinting • Racing
How does it feel? How warm am I? What is my breathing like?				
• No change from resting state • Normal breathing	• Starting to feel warm • Slight increase in breathing rate	• Warmer • Greater increase in breathing rate	• Quite warm • More out of breath	• Very hot/ perspiring heavily • Completely out of breath
	Range needed to stay healthy			

Health Canada, *Handbook for Canada's Physical Activity Guide to Healthy Active Living* (Ottawa, Ont. 1-888-334-9769, http://publications.gc.ca/site/eng/389032/publication.html).

The Borg Perceived Effort Scale: This easy-to-use scale measures an individual's subjective perception of his or her effort. It is an excellent way to assess the intensity of physical activity performed by people taking medications that affect their heart rate. An intensity of 12 or 13 corresponds to a moderate level of effort (*see illustration opposite*). Although the measurement is subjective, an estimate of perceived effort can provide a fairly reliable assessment of the person's actual heart rate during the physical activity.

The Borg scale should be referred to while the physical effort is being performed. The scale ranges from 6 to 20, with 6 corresponding to "no effort at all" and 20 signifying "exhaustion" or "maximal effort". Choose the number that best corresponds to your perception of your effort. It will give you a good idea of the intensity of your physical activity and help you decide if you should speed up or slow down your movements to achieve the intensity you want. Be as honest as possible – the accuracy of your estimate depends on it.

Resistance activities should be started under the supervision of a specialist in physical activity (kinesiologist). He or she can help you set up a program that will let you gradually increase the number of repetitions and modify the type of weights you use.

Diabetes Quebec has produced a video (in French) on this type of activity. It can be found at http://www.diabete.qc.ca/html/activite/enforme/html.

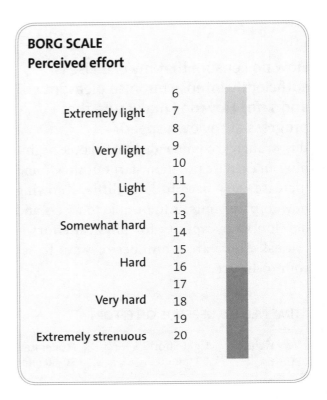

BORG SCALE
Perceived effort

	6
Extremely light	7
	8
Very light	9
	10
Light	11
	12
	13
Somewhat hard	14
	15
Hard	16
	17
Very hard	18
	19
Extremely strenuous	20

When is exercise dangerous for people with diabetes?

In some cases, exercise can be risky. It is contraindicated for people with type 1 diabetes when the diabetes is poorly controlled and blood glucose is:

- lower than 4 mmol/L;
- above 14.0 mmol/L and there are ketone bodies in the urine or blood;
- above 17.0 mmol/L, whether or not there are ketone bodies in the urine or blood.

In some situations, people with diabetes can engage in regular physical activity, but they should always be careful about the types of activities they choose.

For example:

People with diabetes who have heart problems should begin an exercise program only under medical supervision.

People with diabetes who have retinopathy with a risk of hemorrhage should seek medical advice. If an exercise program is approved, options could include swimming, walking and riding a stationary bike instead of anaerobic activities like weightlifting or sports involving blows or jolts (for example, boxing, racket sports such as tennis or badminton, or jogging).

People with diabetes who have serious neuropathy with complete loss of sensation in the feet can do activities such as swimming, biking, rowing on a rowing machine, arm exercises and chair exercises.

Generally speaking, even in special cases like these, short periods of walking remains one of the least risky activities.

People with active wounds on their feet should choose activities that avoid placing pressure on the wounds or that could cause maceration (arm exercises or chair exercises).

What are the potential risks of physical activity for people with diabetes taking certain oral antidiabetic medications or insulin?

People with diabetes who are taking drugs to stimulate the pancreas to produce more insulin (e.g. glyburide, gliclazide, glimepiride, repaglinide) or who are taking insulin run a higher risk of hypoglycemia, especially if the activity is unplanned, prolonged, and of moderate intensity.

It is important to remember that:

- moderate activity sustained for several hours can cause hypoglycemia during the activity but also as long as 12 to 24 hours afterwards. For example, cross-country skiing, major housecleaning or even several hours of shopping can all provoke delayed hypoglycemia;
- the more regular the activity (schedule, duration and intensity), the lower the risk of hypoglycemia.
- very intense physical activity can lead to hyperglycemia.

What precautions should be taken when planning to exercise?

- People with diabetes should measure their blood sugar before any physical activity, whether their treatment is medication to stimulate the pancreas to create more insulin (e.g., glyburide, gliclazide, glimepiride, repaglinide) or insulin.
- The condition of the feet should be checked **before and after** any exercise.
- Alcohol should not be consumed **before, during or after** exercise.
- People with diabetes should always wear a diabetic ID bracelet or pendant.
- People with diabetes should have quickly metabolized carbohydrate sources on hand.
- People taking insulin are advised to use an injection site in a part of the body that will be the least involved in the exercise (e.g., the abdomen).

What can people with diabetes who are taking insulin do to prevent hypoglycemia when exercising?

People with diabetes who are taking rapid- or short-acting insulin before meals need to adapt their treatment to prevent hypoglycemia when exercising.

- When the activity is planned and takes place 1 to 2 hours after a meal, the insulin dose before the meal should be reduced according to the type of exercise, its duration, its intensity, the person's training, and above all, the person's experience.

For example, a man with diabetes who injects 10 units of insulin before a meal plans on taking an hour-long walk at moderate intensity immediately after eating. He can reduce the insulin dose by 75% and inject 2.5 (or 3) units before the meal:

75% x 10 units = 7.5 units

10 units − 7.5 units = 2.5 (or 3) units.

The following table provides an example of how to decrease the pre-meal insulin dose:

INTENSITY OF EFFORT	PERCENTAGE (%) REDUCTION IN THE RAPID- OR SHORT-ACTING INSULIN DOSE, BASED ON DURATION OF EXERCISE	
	30 minutes	60 minutes
Low	25%	50%
Moderate	50%	75%
High	75%	90% to 100%

- When the activity is unplanned and takes place immediately before or after a meal, or when the activity is planned but takes place more than two hours after a meal:

  for blood glucose between 4 mmol/L and 5.5 mmol/L, a carbohydrate snack (15 g to 30 g) is recommended at the beginning of the activity and approximately every 30 to 45 minutes afterward, as long as the activity lasts;

  for blood glucose above 5.5 mmol/L, a snack of about 15 g of carbohydrates is recommended every 30 to 45 minutes while the activity lasts.

Blood glucose should always be measured immediately after exercising to adjust the mounts of insulin and carbohydrates required. In all cases, the need for insulin can decrease after exercise. This sometimes requires reducing the insulin dose for the next meal or at bedtime.

What can people with diabetes do to prevent hypoglycemia when exercising if they are taking oral antidiabetic drugs to stimulate the secretion of insulin?

For people with diabetes who are taking **drugs that stimulate the pancreas to produce insulin (for example, glyburide, gliclazide, glimepiride, repaglinide)**, supplementing carbohydrate intake while exercising can reduce the risks of hypoglycemia. Sometimes – if weight loss is a goal, for example – the dose of the insulin-stimulating drug can be reduced so that additional carbohydrates will not be necessary. This should be done only after discussion with a doctor.

The recommendations are:
for blood glucose between 4.0 mmol/L and 5.5 mmol/L, have a carbohydrate snack (15 g to 30 g) at the beginning of the activity and then approximately every 30 to 45 minutes afterwards, as long as the activity lasts; **for blood glucose above 5.5 mmol/L**, carbohydrate supplementation is required only if hypoglycemia occurs during exercise.

If supplementation is needed, have a snack of about 15 g of carbohydrates every 30 to 45 minutes during the activity. Be sure to check blood glucose levels before eating to avoid overeating.

The following chart is a guide to adding carbohydrates during exercise. Carbohydrate supplementation is especially useful during unplanned exercise and almost always neces-

TYPE OF EXERCISE	BLOOD GLUCOSE (MMOL/L)	CARBOHYDRATE SUPPLEMENTATION
Short duration (< 30 min) at light intensity	≤ 5.5 > 5.5	10 g to 15 g not necessary
Moderate duration (30 to 60 min) at Moderate intensity	≤ 5.5 5.5 - 9.9 10.0 - 13.9	30 g to 45 g 15 g every 30 to 45 min of exercise not necessary
Long duration (> 60 min) at elevated intensity	≤ 5.5 5.5 - 9.9 > 9.9	45 g 30 g to 45 g 15 g every hour

Adapted from : Hayes, C. *J. Am. Diet Assoc.* 97 (Suppl 2) : S167-S171, 1997

sary during exercise that lasts a long time or is quite intense and results in a significant expenditure of energy.

If you frequently experience hypoglycemia after engaging in physical activity, you are strongly urged to see your doctor.

What precautions should be taken by people with diabetes who take insulin or oral antidiabetic drugs that stimulate the secretion of insulin?

People with diabetes treated with insulin or oral antidiabetic drugs that stimulate the secretion of insulin should:

- always measure blood glucose before, during and after an exercise session, and more often than normal in the 24 hours following prolonged physical activity;
- always carry foods containing carbohydrates to correct hypoglycemia.

CLASS OF DRUG	RISK OF HYPOGLYCEMIA
Biguanides (e.g., metformine)	No
Glucosidase inhibitors (e.g., acarbose)	No
DPP-4 inhibitors (e.g., sitagliptine)	No
Thiazolidinediones (e.g., pioglitazone)	No
Sulfonylureas (e.g., glyburide)	Yes
Meglitinides (e.g., repaglinide)	Yes
Insulin	Yes

* If you are taking medication associated with a risk of hypoglyemia, talk to your doctor to determine how to adjust the medication or your carbohydrate consumption when you exercise.

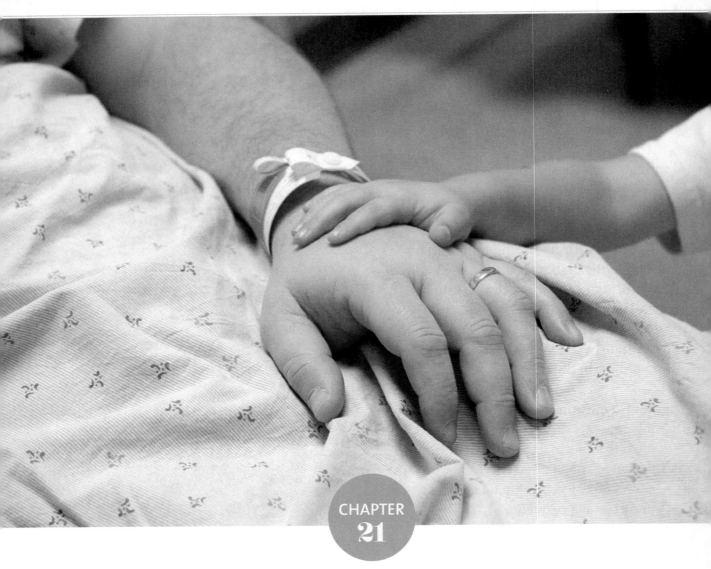

CHAPTER
21

Hyperglycemic Emergencies:

Diabetic Acidosis and the Hyperosmolar State

What hyperglycemic emergencies arise in people with diabetes?

Two types of hyperglycemic emergency can affect people with diabetes. They are:

- diabetic acidosis;
- hyperosmolar states.

These two conditions are caused by a lack of insulin. Diabetic acidosis is more common in people with type 1 diabetes, while **hyperosmolar states occur primarily in people with type 2 diabetes**, usually when they are older. However, both conditions are possible in people with either type 1 or type 2 diabetes.

What is diabetic acidosis?

Diabetic acidosis is caused by a lack of insulin. It is characterized by hyperglycemia and an accumulation of ketone bodies in the blood. This makes the blood acidic and can lead to **extreme fatigue**, **abdominal pains**, **nausea** and **vomiting**. Diabetic acidosis also gives the breath a fruity odour and causes intense thirst as well as deep and rapid breathing. In some cases, it provokes disorientation and confusion. If left untreated, it can result in a coma and potentially death.

What causes diabetic acidosis?

Diabetic acidosis is always caused by a **shortage of insulin** in the blood. When there is insufficient insulin, glucose cannot enter certain cells of the body and accumulates in the blood. The body is then forced to draw on its fat reserves for energy. The **breakdown of fats** causes the liver to produce ketone bodies. The ketone bodies, which are acids, then accumulate in the blood and spill over into the urine.

Diabetic acidosis may be a sign of type 1 diabetes.

Factors that can bring on this complication of diabetes are:

- the omission of certain insulin injections, inadequate dose adjustment, or an insulin pump malfunction;
- situations increasing the need for insulin (infection, myocardial infarction, acute abdominal disease, trauma, hyperthyroidism, medications such as cortisone or atypical antipsychotics, some drugs, especially cocaine, and significant stress).

How is diabetic acidosis detected?

Diabetic acidosis is detected by the **presence of ketone bodies** in the urine or blood, along with elevated blood glucose levels, often higher than **20 mmol/L**.

How can people with type 1 diabetes avoid diabetic acidosis?

Generally, diabetic acidosis can be avoided by taking the following precautions:

- **Check blood glucose levels regularly** and more frequently during illness or in times of exceptional stress.
- If blood glucose is **higher than 14 mmol/L**, check for ketone bodies in the urine (use Chemstrip uG/K®, Keto-Diastix® or Ketostix® test strips) or the level of ketone bodies in a blood sample from the fingertip (use Nova Max® Plus™ reader or Precision Xtra® strips).
- Follow a dietician-recommended meal plan.
- Take insulin as prescribed.
- Follow the doctor's instructions for insulin doses on sick days when a normal diet is impossible.

A number of methods can be used to determine the proper correction dose for days when you are ill. It is very important to draw up a personal action plan with your doctor so that you know what additional doses to take, as well as when and under what circumstances you should take them.

Correction doses use the same insulin as the type used for meals (rapid or short-acting)

Call the doctor or go to the emergency room if one of the following five situations occurs:

- blood glucose is higher than 20 mmol/L;
- the ketosis reading (ketone bodies) in the urine is moderate (4 mmol/L) or high (8 mmol/L –16 mmol/L) (*See page 201*);
- the ketosis level reading from the fingertip is higher than 3 mmol/L (*See page 201*);
- you are vomiting continually and cannot retain liquids;
- the following conditions persist despite treatment: extreme fatigue, weakness, dizziness, abdominal pains, nausea and vomiting, fruity breath odour, intense thirst, fast and heavy breathing.

What is a hyperosmolar state?

A hyperosmolar state usually occurs in people with **type 2 diabetes** who develop an **increased resistance to insulin**. Insulin resistance prevents **glucose** from entering the cells properly, leading to its **accumulation in the blood**.

If kidney function is impaired, it is more difficult to eliminate excess sugar in the blood through the urine. Sugar can therefore accumulate in the blood until it reaches very high levels (above 30mmol/L), especially if not enough fluids are ingested. Although there is very little insulin in the blood at this point, it is usually sufficient to prevent the breakdown of fats, and diabetic acidosis does not generally develop.

In a hyperosmolar state, blood glucose levels rise, causing extreme fatigue and thirst (although some elderly people do not feel thirst). Frequent and profuse urination also occurs, leading to dehydration. This can be followed by a drop in blood pressure and in some cases disorientation, which can lead to coma and, if left untreated, even death.

What causes a hyperosmolar state?

A hyperosmolar state is always caused by a shortage of insulin in the blood. Because a small amount of insulin remains, however, ketone bodies do not form and diabetic acidosis does not develop.

A hyperosmolar glycemic state newly diagnosed may be indicative of unrecognised type 2 diabetes.

This complication of diabetes can occur:
- if antidiabetic drugs (pills or injection) or insulin are skipped;
- in situations that create an increased need for insulin, for example in the case of infection, myocardial infarction, acute abdominal disease, trauma, hyperthyroidism, the use of medications such as cortisone, diuretics, lithium, or atypical antipsychotics, the use of drugs (especially cocaine), and significant stress.

Some of the time, a hyperosmolar state occurs in people who do not feel thirst or who are unable to hydrate themselves, which is sometimes the case for elderly people or individuals who have lost autonomy.

How is a hyperosmolar state detected?

The symptoms of a hyperosmolar state can include intense thirst, frequent and profuse urination over several days, and especially, blood glucose levels over 30 mmol/L. There is usually no accumulation of ketone bodies in the blood or urine.

How can a hyperosmolar state be avoided?

The following tips can generally help a person avoid a hyperosmolar state:

- Measure blood glucose levels regularly and do so more frequently during illness or in times of exceptional stress.
- Stay hydrated; drink 250 mL of water every hour if blood glucose levels are high or if high blood glucose causes an increased amount and frequency of urination.
- Follow a dietician-recommended meal plan.
- Take antidiabetic drugs (pills or injections) or insulin as prescribed.
- Follow the recommendations of the doctor and dietician concerning the appropriate nutrients to consume in solid and liquid form and the dosages of antidiabetic drug (pills or injections) or insulin to take when illness makes it impossible to follow a normal diet.
- Do not quench thirst with fruit juice or regular pop.

Call your doctor or go to the emergency room if one of the following four situations occurs:

- blood glucose is higher than 30 mmol/L;
- you have heart or kidney failure that requires you to limit your intake of liquids;
- an illness makes normal nutrition and especially liquid intake impossible;
- the following conditions persist despite treatment: extreme fatigue, intense thirst, frequent and profuse urination, abnormal breathing.

IN SUMMARY

The action you take depends on:

your blood sugar;

whether or not there are ketone bodies in your urine or blood;

you are showing signs or symptoms.

SUGGESTED APPROACH TO THE DETECTION AND TREATMENT OF DIABETIC ACIDOSIS AND/OR HYPEROSMOLAR STATES

Blood glucose (mmol/L)	Ketosis level reading (mmol/L) in the urine (with Keto-Diastix® or Ketostix® strips or in the blood (with Precision Xtra® strips)	Symptoms	Suggested action
13 - 14	• None or trace • Urine: 0.5 • Blood: less than 0.6	• Frequent urination • Intense thirst	• Drink 250 mL of water every hour • Measure blood glucose levels every 6 hours
14 - 20	• Low • Urine: 1.5 • Blood: 0.6 to 1.5	• Frequent urination • Intense thirst	• Drink 250 mL of water every hour • Measure blood glucose levels every 4 hours • Adjust insulin doses according to doctor's recommendations • Or call your doctor
14 - 20	• Medium • Urine: 4 • Blood: 1.5 to 3	• Frequent urination • Intense thirst • Nausea • Vomiting • Abdominal pain (diarrhea)	• Measure blood glucose and ketone bodies every 4 hours • Immediately adjust your insulin dose according to doctor's recommendations for sick days • Call your doctor or go to the hospital if there is no improvement
Above 20	• Medium to high • Urine: 8 to 16 • Blood: higher than 3	• Nausea • Vomiting • Abdominal pain (diarrhea) • Fruity breath	• Go to the hospital: This is diabetic acidosis
Above 30	• None or low • Urine: 0 to 1.5 • Blood: 0 to 0.6	• Frequent urination • Intense thirst • Extreme weakness	• Go to the hospital: This is a hyperosmolar state

Check urinary ketone body levels with Chemstrip uG/K® test strips. Follow instructions in the product insert.
Check blood ketone body levels with the Nova Max® Plus™ reader. Follow instructions in the product insert.

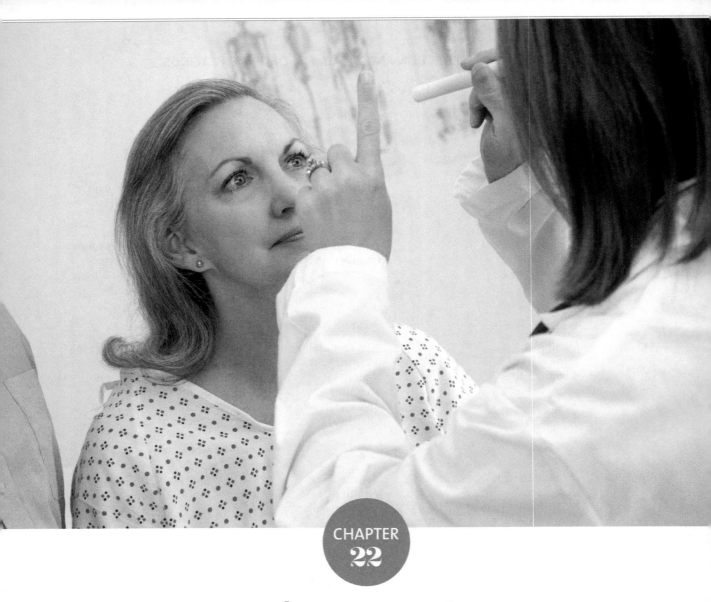

Chronic Complications

What are the potential long-term complications of diabetes?

If blood glucose levels are not well managed, after a number of years the risk of certain complications increases. They can affect:

- **the eyes** (diabetic retinopathy);
- **the kidneys** (diabetic nephropathy);
- **the nerves** (diabetic neuropathy);
- **the heart and blood vessels** (cardiac or peripheral atherosclerosis).

How can diabetes affect the eyes?

Over time, hyperglycemia can cause **changes to the small vessels at the back of the eye**, potentially compromising blood circulation and causing hemorrhage: this is called **diabetic retinopathy**. Inadequate treatment of diabetes and retinopathy can lead to blindness. Diabetic retinopathy is the leading cause of blindness in the 20 to 64 year old age group.

When should I get my eyes checked?

If your vision is affected. Some people see spider webs or spots in their field of vision.
If your vision is not affected. Often the changes at the back of the eye do not cause any vision problems.

It is therefore **very important to visit an ophthalmologist or an optometrist regularly**. The examination will involve dilation of the pupil to better view the retina. Special digital cameras that take photos of the back of the eye can also be used to detect abnormalities. If any are found, the diagnosis must be confirmed in an examination by an ophthalmologist.

People with type 1 diabetes are advised to consult an ophthalmologist or optometrist five years after diagnosis and once a year after that. People with type 2 diabetes should see an ophthalmologist or optometrist at the time of diagnosis and then every year or two years after. If there are any signs of damage to the eyes, however, people with either type of diabetes should see an ophthalmologist more frequently.

Temporary changes in vision (blurriness) can result from variations in blood glucose levels. **Hyperglycemia and hypoglycemia can cause blurry vision**, but it is corrected when blood glucose is normalized.

What should I do to protect my eyes?

Protect your eyes by:

- keeping **blood glucose levels** as close to normal as possible;
- seeing an **ophthalmologist** or **optometrist** regularly;
- controlling your **blood pressure**;
- **quitting smoking**, if applicable.

What are the potential long-term effects of diabetes on the kidneys?

In the long term, hyperglycemia can cause changes in the **small blood vessels of the kidneys**, hampering their blood filtration and purification functions: this is called **diabetic nephropathy**. If diabetes is not properly controlled, this condition can develop into complete loss of renal function. In such a case, dialysis (artificial kidney) or a kidney transplant is necessary. Diabetes is the main cause of dialysis in the Western world.

How do I know if diabetes has caused kidney damage?

The only way to detect whether diabetes has had any effect on the kidneys is through a laboratory analysis to detect **microalbuminuria** (small amounts of albumin in the urine). A **microalbuminuria** screening test, which requires nothing more than a urine sample, should be performed at the time of diagnosis of type 2 diabetes and five years after diagnosis of type 1 diabetes, after which the screening should be repeated once a year. In some cases, the doctor will ask for urine samples spanning a 24-hour period to better assess the severity of the nephropathy. A rise in blood pressure can also signal the onset of kidney damage.

What should I do to protect my kidneys?

Protect your kidneys by:

- keeping **blood glucose levels** as close to normal as possible;
- checking for **albumin** in the urine once a year;
- checking **blood pressure** regularly and treating high blood pressure aggressively;
- **quitting smoking**, if applicable;
- **taking drugs** to slow the progress of the nephropathy. These are the same drugs used to control blood pressure and treat heart failure. The doctor may suggest them if indicated.

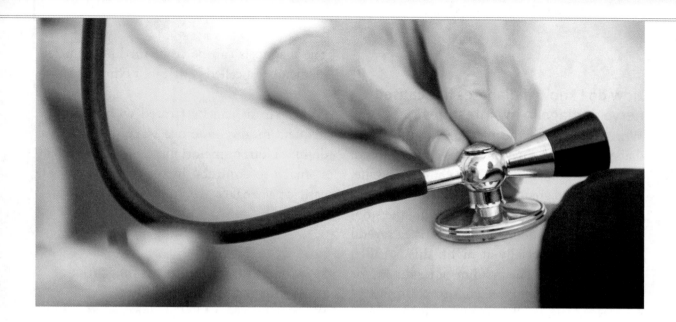

What are the potential long-term effects of diabetes on the nerves?

Over the long term, hyperglycemia can cause **nerve damage**, particularly in the extremities but also in organs such as the intestines, stomach, bladder, heart and genitals. This is known as **diabetic neuropathy**.

How do I know if diabetes has caused nerve damage in my extremities?

In most cases, nerve damage manifests as **a decrease in sensitivity to pain, heat and cold in the extremities**. Another sign is a burning sensation or neuropathic pain. The diagnosis can be confirmed by your doctor or through a special test called electromyography (EMG). This type of complication is also known as "per-

ipheral diabetic neuropathy" and affects the lower limbs more often than the upper limbs.

If the symptoms of neuropathic pain are incapacitating, appropriate treatment is prescribed (*see chapter 23*).

What is the biggest danger of nerve damage in the extremities?

(*see chapter 23*)

The biggest danger of a loss of sensation, particularly in the feet, is **unperceived self-injury** (from ill-fitting shoes, hot water, a needle, etc.). Such an injury can become infected and, if circulation is compromised, can lead to gangrene and amputation.

How do I know if diabetes has caused nerve damage in my intestines?

When the nerves in the intestines are affected by diabetes, stool evacuation can be compromised: this is called **constipation**. In an advanced state, when stools stagnate in the colon, normal intestinal bacteria can multiply, liquefying the stool and triggering sudden, intense diarrhea several times a day, especially at night: this is called **diabetic diarrhea**. The first line of treatment for constipation is diet. Fibre consumption should be increased gradually and plenty of water consumed. Fibre supplements in capsules or powder form (e.g. Metamucil®) can make the stool firmer and help with evacuation. If fibre and water are not sufficient, constipation can be treated with laxatives such as docusate sodium or sennosides. Diabetic diarrhea can also be treated with antibiotics such as tetracycline or erythromycin. Sometimes, anti-diarrheal agents such as loperamide or diphenoxylate are also required.

How do I know if diabetes has caused nerve damage in my stomach?

When the nerves of the stomach are affected, the stomach empties more slowly: this is **diabetic gastroparesis**. This usually manifests as a feeling of bloating and/or regurgitation after a meal. Food absorption becomes irregular, which can make it more difficult to control blood glucose (hyperglycemia and hypoglycemia).

The diagnosis can be confirmed by a nuclear medicine test called gastric emptying.

Gastroparesis can be treated with small and frequent meals and, if necessary, drugs such as domperidone or metoclopramide that cause the stomach to contract. In very serious cases, a gastric pacemaker may improve symptoms.

How do I know if diabetes has caused nerve damage in my bladder?

When the nerves of the bladder are affected by diabetes, it is more difficult to sense when the bladder is full and the bladder does not empty completely during urination: this is called **neurogenic bladder**. It can result in loss of urine due to overflow and, if urine stagnates in the bladder, a risk of a urinary tract infection that can extend to the kidneys. Neurogenic bladder can be diagnosed with an echography of the bladder after urination to determine whether there is any urine retention. Regular urination while exerting pressure on the bladder can help avoid urine overflow. In the case of significant urine retention, drugs that help the bladder to contract such as betanechol can be used.

Nerve damage to the bladder can also manifest as hyperactive bladder, which has the following symptoms:
- increased frequency of urination;
- urgency of urination;
- urinary incontinence.

This condition results from nerve damage causing a signal to be sent to the bladder to contract at inappropriate times. Drugs such as oxybutinin (Ditropan®, Oxytrol®) can help control these symptoms.

How do I know if diabetes has caused nerve damage in my heart?

Most of the time, nerve damage in the heart is asymptomatic, although in some cases it can cause accelerated heartbeat (tachycardia) and/or arrhythmia. There is no specific treatment. In cases of persistent accelerated heartbeat, beta-blockers such as metoprolol or atenolol can be prescribed.

How does a man know if diabetes has caused nerve damage in his genital organs?

Nerve damage in the male genitalia causes difficulty achieving and maintaining erection, thus making sexual intercourse challenging or impossible. This is known as **erectile dysfunction**. It can be treated with certain oral medications such as Viagra®, Cialis® or Levitra®. In some cases, local treatments such as prostaglandin are necessary, either introduced through the urethra (urinary duct) in the form of suppositories (for example, Muse®) or injected into the base of the penis (for example, Caverject®).

What should I do to prevent nerve damage and its complications?

Prevent nerve damage and its complications by:
- keeping **blood glucose levels** as close to normal as possible;
- inspecting the feet daily, taking measures to avoid **trauma to the feet**, and seeing a doctor in the event of even the slightest injury (*see chapter 23*);
- reporting any **digestive problems**;
- reporting any **bladder problems**;
- reporting any incidence of **erectile dysfunction**;
- reporting any incidence of **accelerated or irregular heartbeat**;
- seeking aggressive treatment for **high blood pressure**.

How does diabetes damage the heart and blood vessels?

Diabetes can cause damage to the heart and blood vessels by accelerating the aging of the arteries (hardening of the arteries) and the process of **atherosclerosis**, in which artery walls are thickened and arteries become blocked with atheroma (plaque consisting of fats, blood cells, and inflammatory cells). This can block circulation in parts of the body such as the heart, lower limbs, or even the brain. Damage to the blood vessels of the heart is the primary cause of morbidity and death in people with diabetes.

What are the potential complications of damage to the heart and blood vessels?

Complications depend on the part of the body affected:

- if there is damage to the heart, potential complications include angina, **myocardial infarction**, heart failure, or arrhythmia;
- if there is damage to the brain, potential complications include **stroke, which can cause paralysis, speech impairment**, or dizziness;
- if there is damage to the lower limbs, potential complications include **pain when walking, gangrene, or even amputation**.

How do I know if diabetes has caused damage to my heart and blood vessels?

There are signs that can reveal atherosclerosis and circulation problems:

- **chest pain** and/or **difficulty breathing** during physical exertion;
- **pain in the calves** when walking (claudication).

In some cases, however, atherosclerosis is asymptomatic, particularly in its early stages, and is diagnosed only through a medical exam or special tests such as a resting or exercise electrocardiogram (EKG or ECG), an exercise echocardiogram, a heart scan, cardiac scintigraphy (MIBI), or a Doppler test (using ultrasound to examine the state of blood vessels) of the blood vessels in the neck or the lower limbs.

What should I do to prevent diabetes from damaging my heart and blood vessels?

Reduce the risk of damage to the heart and blood vessels by:

- keeping **blood glucose levels** as close to normal as possible, especially in the years following diagnosis of diabetes;
- checking **blood pressure** regularly and treating high blood pressure aggressively;
- avoiding **saturated fats** (especially of animal origin) as much as possible;
- having **blood lipid levels** checked regularly and treating any abnormalities aggressively;

- **quitting smoking**, if applicable;
- **exercising**;
- taking an aspirin every day if you have ever suffered from cardiovascular disease. A daily aspirin is no longer systematically recommended for people with diabetes who do not have cardiovascular disease; the doctor will tell you if it is required.

What is high blood pressure?

In the general population, blood pressure is considered high if it is 140/90 or higher. People with diabetes are urged to follow stricter standards, however. Blood pressure is considered high if it is greater than or equal to 130/80 in a person with diabetes.

Why should people with diabetes treat high blood pressure aggressively?

High blood pressure significantly increases the complications of diabetes that can damage the eyes, nerves, kidneys, heart and blood vessels.

It has been clearly shown that treating high blood pressure in people with diabetes significantly decreases the development and progression of complications associated with the disease.

When and why should people with diabetes begin blood lipid treatment?

Blood lipids – particularly LDL ("bad") cholesterol – are major risk factors for cardiovascular disease. Since people with diabetes run a higher risk of heart and blood vessel disease, their LDL cholesterol levels should be lower than those in people without diabetes. Studies have shown that statin therapy can reduce the onset of disease of the heart and blood vessels in people with diabetes.

According to the 2013 recommendations of the Canadian Diabetes Association, the following people should receive statin therapy:
- anyone with diabetes over the age of 40;
- anyone with diabetes who has had cardiovascular complications in the past, regardless of age;
- anyone with diabetes who also has retinopathy, nephropathy, or neuropathy, regardless of age;
- anyone with diabetes over the age of 30, with no known complications, who has had evolving diabetes for over 15 years.

The objective is to achieve a level of LDL cholesterol below 2 mmol/L or a 50% reduction of the current level.

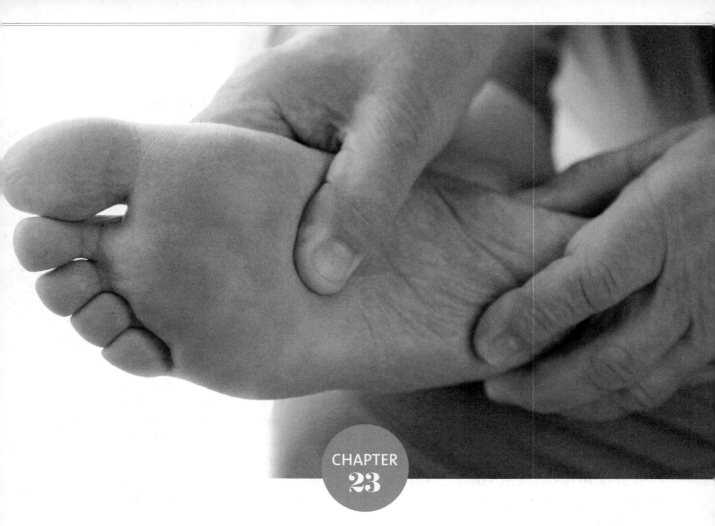

Foot Care and General Hygiene

Why is diabetic foot a public health issue?

Diabetic foot – complications of diabetes affecting the foot – is a major public health issue because it is the primary cause of non-trauma-related amputation. In the long term, poorly controlled diabetes is associated with peripheral neuropathy, especially of the feet, the symptoms of which include loss of sensitivity to touch, pain, heat and cold. As a result of this loss of sensitivity, people with diabetes can injure themselves without noticing. A small wound can become infected, and if the person already has circulatory problems, gangrene can develop, possibly requiring amputation. Proper foot care can prevent 80% of these amputations. It is therefore a very important issue.

What problems can lead to diabetic foot complications in people with diabetes?

The feet of people with diabetes are more fragile than those of people who do not have the disease. Over time, hyperglycemia can lead to the following foot problems:

- **nerve damage** resulting in loss of sensitivity to touch, pain, heat and cold;
- **a tendency for the skin to become thinner and drier,** to become more easily irritated, and to develop calluses (hyperkeratosis) at pressure points;

- a tendency for **the arteries to thicken and harden,** resulting in reduced circulation in the feet;
- **a susceptibility to infection** because the body is less able to defend itself against microbes when blood glucose levels are high.

How should I examine my feet?

The responsibility for foot care should be shared between the health care team and the person with diabetes. If you have diabetes, do the following:

- examine your feet closely every day after a bath or shower;
- under a good light source, sit down and examine both feet from every angle (top, bottom, and between the toes);
- use a mirror to examine the soles of the feet if you lack the flexibility to see them otherwise;
- if your vision is impaired or if you cannot reach your feet with your hands, ask another person to help you;
- follow up the self-exam with a thorough professional examination every time you visit a doctor, podiatrist, or nurse specializing in foot care.

What should I look for?

Look carefully for:

1 **lesions between the toes** caused by fungi that thrive in humid conditions (athlete's foot);

2 **calluses:** heavily callused skin (often located under the foot) can make the skin fragile and provides a good place for microbes to multiply;

3 **corns:**
   - on the toes, produced by friction with shoes;
   - between the toes, known as "soft corns" (or "kissing corns"), caused by the toes being compressed together;

4 **cracks:** crevices in callused skin (often on or around the heel) are particularly well-suited for microbial growth. Excess callused skin can always be traced to a specific cause:
   - poor foot posture (position, compression); see your doctor as soon as possible;
   - the use of methods that can harm the feet: razor blades, knives, graters or corn-removal preparations; these products and instruments should be avoided;
   - foreign bodies in the shoes or seams that can injure the feet; check by running your hand along the inside of your shoes.

What are the first signs of foot problems?

The feet should also be examined for the following problems:
- changes in skin colour, unusual redness;
- unusually high skin temperature;
- swollen feet or ankles;
- pain in the legs or feet;
- ingrown toenails;
- toenail fungus;
- open sores that heal slowly;
- calluses that bleed or appear to be infected;
- dry and fissured skin, especially around the heel;
- scratches;
- bunions;
- warts;
- loss of sensation in the feet.

How can a person with diabetes reduce the risk of foot problems?

To limit the risk of developing foot problems:

- keep blood glucose as close to normal as possible;
- quit smoking, if applicable;
- lose weight, if necessary;
- reduce alcohol consumption, if applicable;
- get regular exercise;
- see a doctor, podiatrist, nurse specialized in foot care, or any other specialist, as needed.

What are the top-ten foot care suggestions for people with diabetes?

1 **Examine your feet every day**, asking for help from family and friends if needed:

- Examine your feet closely all over, looking for lesions, cuts or any malformation.
- Regularly check the sensitivity of your feet (on a schedule recommended by your doctor):
- Put a dry pea in your shoe and walk a few steps to see whether you can feel the foreign body; remove the pea immediately to avoid causing injury.

2 **Never go barefoot**, not even in the house, and especially not on a beach or in any public area:

- Put on slippers when you get out of bed.
- Wear comfortable shoes during the day.

3 **Wash your feet every day:**

- Check the water temperature with your wrist, elbow or a thermometer; the water should be lukewarm (below 37ºC).
- Wash your feet with mild soap (e.g., unscented Dove®, Aveeno®, Cetaphil®, Neutrogena®, Keri®, etc.).
- Avoid soaking your feet for longer than 10 minutes to avoid maceration and softening of the skin.
- Dry your feet carefully, especially between and under the toes; humidity encourages the development of fungi (e.g., athlete's foot).

4 **Be sure the skin is completely dry:**

- Apply a thin layer of neutral (unscented) moisturizing cream (for example, Nivea®, Lubriderm®, Vaseline Intensive Care®, Glycerodermine®, etc.), except between the toes.
- Once or twice a week after a bath or shower, use a moistened pumice stone to rub areas where there is hyperkeratosis (thickening of the skin). Avoid rubbing back and forth, and use long, continuous movements in one direction. Never use a metal grater, as this can cause injury.

5 **Avoid cutting your toenails too short:**

- Nails should be filed straight across, a little longer than the tips of the toes, and the corners filed after a bath or shower. This will prevent you from developing ingrown toenails and from injuring yourself.
- Nails should be filed instead of a clipped or cut; this will help avoid injury.
- Handle round-ended scissors and nail clippers with care. Anyone lacking in dexterity or suffering from impaired or reduced vision should avoid using them altogether;
- Never tear your toenails.

6 **Never self-treat for calluses, corns or blisters:**

- Avoid so-called "bathroom surgery": never use pointed scissors, sharp clippers, razor blades, lancets, scalpels, or metal files to remove a corn.
- Never use over-the-counter solutions or plasters with a salicylic acid base, since they can cause skin necrosis.
- See a foot care specialist, taking care to tell him or her that you have diabetes.

7 **Change your socks every day:**

- Wear clean socks (or stockings), and wash them every day.
- Wear socks that fit. Be sure they are loose and long enough and do not squeeze the toes. Avoid wearing tight socks that leave marks on the calves and cut off circulation.
- Avoid thick stitching; if the socks have seams, wear them inside out.
- Avoid shoes with holes or patches that create points of friction.
- Wear socks that keep the feet dry, made with a blend of cotton and synthetic fibres (acrylic, orlon, polypropylene, Coolmax, etc.). People who sweat a lot should avoid socks that contain nylon.

8 **Choose your shoes carefully:**

- Always wear socks with shoes.
- Choose shoes fastened with laces, buckles or velcro; they should be made from supple leather or canvas and roomy enough to let the toes move.
- Choose non-skid soles.
- Buy shoes late in the afternoon; because your feet will be swollen, it will be easier to choose shoes that fit correctly.
- Break in new shoes gradually by wearing them for half a day at first.
- Carefully inspect the inside of your shoes before wearing them; run your hand along the inside to feel for any foreign bodies or seams that could injure your feet.
- Avoid pointy shoes and shoes with high heels (over 3 cm).

9 **Watch out for burns or frostbite:**
- If your feet are cold, wear socks, even in bed. Avoid hot-water bottles, electric blankets and hot water.
- Use sunscreen with at least 15 SPF to lower the risk of sunburn.
- Never use powerful products or irritants (for example, chlorine bleach or other types of bleach).
- Make sure the skin is covered, especially in winter, when the weather is cold and dry.

10 **Immediately contact** your foot care specialist (doctor, podiatrist or nurse) if you notice any discoloration, loss of sensation or a lesion.

Everyone with diabetes should have a foot examination by a medical professional at least twice a year. People at higher risk should have more frequent exams.

Which moisturizing creams should a person with diabetes use for foot care?

If your skin tends to be dry, use a daily moisturizer, preferably an unscented product without coloring. Avoid applying it between your toes to avoid maceration. Apply a thin layer of cream after a bath or shower.

There are three main kinds of moisturizing products:
- **hydrating products with humectants**, which soften the skin and diminish fine lines (e.g., Nivea®, Glycerodermine®, Glaxal Base®, Aquatain®, Complex-15®, etc.);
- **anti-dehydration products**, which reduce the evaporation of moisture by creating a film on the skin (e.g., Moisturel®, Lubriderm® (Lotion), Cetaphil®, Aveeno® (Lotion), Keri® (Lotion), Vaseline Intensive Care® (Lotion), Neutrogena®, Aquaphor®, Prevex®, Barrier Creme®, Akildia®, Curel®, Eucrin®, Elta®, etc.);
- **hydrating products with keratolytic and exfoliating properties**, which help remove dead skin cells. These products should be **used with care and be applied only on the stratum-corneum (top layer) of the skin.** Urea may cause a burning or tingling sensation on dry or cracked skin (e.g., Uremol-10®, Uremol-20®, Dermal Therapy® at 10%, 15%, 20% or 25% urea, Lacticare® Lotion, Lac-Hydrin® Lotion, Urisec®, etc.)..

Which antiseptic products should a person with diabetes use for sores or lesions on the feet?

Wash the sore with water and mild soap, then rinse and dry it well.

1 **Disinfect the skin with an antiseptic** (according to a doctor's recommendations):
   - 70% alcohol swab;
   - Proviodine swab;
   - 0.05% chlorhexidine gluconate (e.g., Hibidil®, Baxedin®).

2 **If there is inflammation,** apply a compress soaked in physiological saline solution three or four times a day. Watch for signs of infection over the next 24 to 48 hours. Avoid using adhesive tape directly on the skin. If redness worsens or if there is pus, see a doctor immediately.

3 **If your doctor recommends foot baths,** use one of the following products in one litre of lukewarm boiled water for no longer than 10 minutes:
   - 15 ml (1 tbsp.) of Proviodine®;
   - 15 ml (1 tbsp.) of Hibitane® 4% (chlorhexidine gluconate 4%);
   - 30 ml (2 tbsp.) of Hibitane® 2% (chlorhexidine gluconate 2%).

Wash your feet again under running water and dry them well, especially between the toes. See a doctor if the sore does not heal.

It is important to discover the cause of the problem so that it is does not recur.

How can circulation in the feet be improved?

There are a number of simple, readily available methods to improve circulation and maintain or improve the flexibility of the feet.

1 Do not smoke.
2 Do not cross your legs when sitting.
3 Keep moving – do not remain standing or sitting in one place for too long.
4 Walk as much as you can, within your limits and abilities.
5 When seated, rest your legs on a footstool whenever possible.
6 Do foot exercises regularly – repeat each one 20 times:
   - put a towel on the floor and try to pick it up with your toes;
   - stand on the tips of your toes, then lower your body weight down onto your heels; use a support if necessary (be careful not to fall);
   - flex your ankle, pointing your feet up and down;
   - rotate your feet, first in one direction, then the other;
   - rock in an armchair, pushing with your toes.

What is diabetic neuropathic pain?

The term "diabetic neuropathy" refers to nerve disease associated with diabetes. The term neuropathic pain describes pain caused by nerve damage.

What are the symptoms of diabetic neuropathic pain?

People with diabetes suffering from neuropathic pain use many different terms to describe it, some not necessarily related to pain. Neuropathic pain may be accompanied by:

- burning sensations;
- numbness;
- stinging;
- tingling;
- a feeling of electric shock;
- sensitivity to touch or cold;
- formication;
- a feeling of being crushed;
- deep, shooting pains;
- a feeling of walking on cotton wool.

How is diabetic neuropathic pain treated?

People with diabetes can lower the risk of developing neuropathic complications by properly managing their blood sugar levels. In some cases, proper control of diabetes, physical exercise, meal plans and relaxation exercises combined with drug treatment can help reduce pain. Your doctor may prescribe medications such as amitriptyline, gabapentine (Neurontin®), duloxetine (Cymblata®) or pregabaline (Lyrica®).

What are neuropathic ulcers?

A neuropathic ulcer is a sore or wound on the foot resulting from neuropathy. It develops on pressure points on the bottom of the foot due to calluses or foot deformations. In many cases, people with diabetes continue to walk around despite such foot injuries because they lack sensitivity in their feet, unwittingly making them worse. In some cases, a sore develops in the middle of a callus, possibly worsening and becoming infected, especially if blood glucose is poorly controlled. If the ulcer does not receive adequate treatment, it can become gangrenous and amputation may be necessary.

If you are concerned in any way about a sore on your foot, see your doctor as quickly as possible. Foot ulcers will heal with the appropriate treatment.

Why is dental hygiene particularly important for people with diabetes?

People with diabetes should manage their dental health with as much care as their skin or feet. There are two major reasons:

- Poorly controlled diabetes causes a high risk of cavities, gum sores or infection.
- Any infection can raise blood glucose levels and hamper the control of diabetes.

What are the main types of oral lesions?

Cavities

Cavities destroy teeth. The main cause of cavities is dental plaque, a whitish deposit that sticks to the enamel. The formation of dental plaque is encouraged by sweet foods, failure to brush the teeth and gums, and alcohol, which reduces acidity levels in the mouth.

Gingivitis

Gingivitis is caused by the deposit of bacteria that create plaque between the teeth and gums. The gum becomes bright red, inflamed and swollen, and tends to bleed if touched.

Periodontitis

Periodontitis develops if gingivitis remains untreated. The germs along the roots of the affected teeth multiply, and the inflammation spreads to areas deep within the gums and the bone supporting the teeth. The teeth become loose and can even fall out painlessly.

What kind of dental hygiene measures should people with diabetes practice?

The main preventive dental hygiene measures are:

- Maintain blood glucose levels as close to normal as possible.
- Brush your teeth carefully after every meal.
- Use dental floss every day.
- See a dentist twice a year, or more often if necessary.
- See a denturologist once every five years to adjust dental prostheses, if necessary.
- Drink alcohol in moderation, so as not to reduce acidity in the mouth.
- Do not smoke.

People with diabetes should always inform the health professionals they consult that they have diabetes. In the event of any kind of medical procedure, antibiotics may be prescribed to prevent infection.

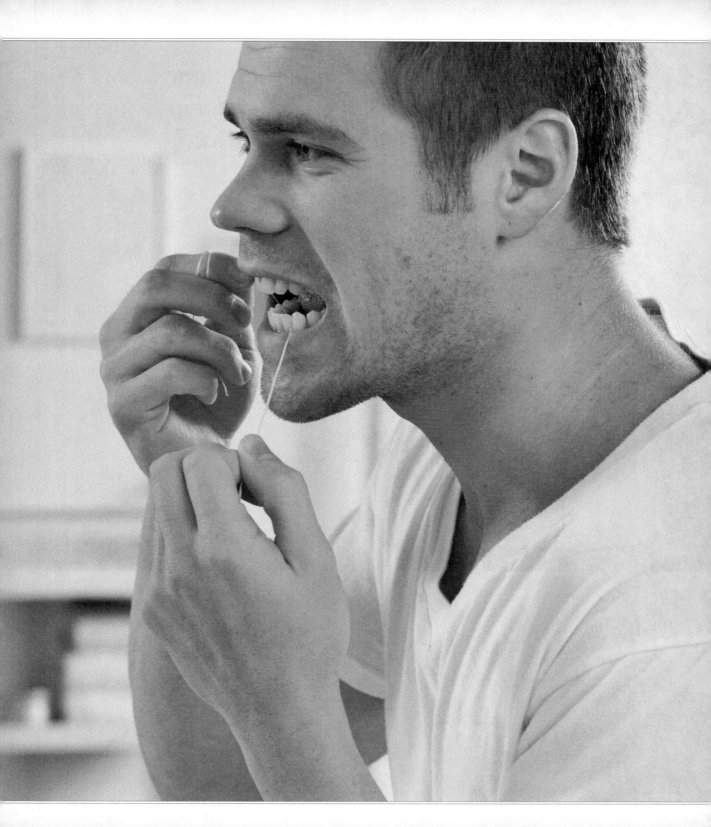

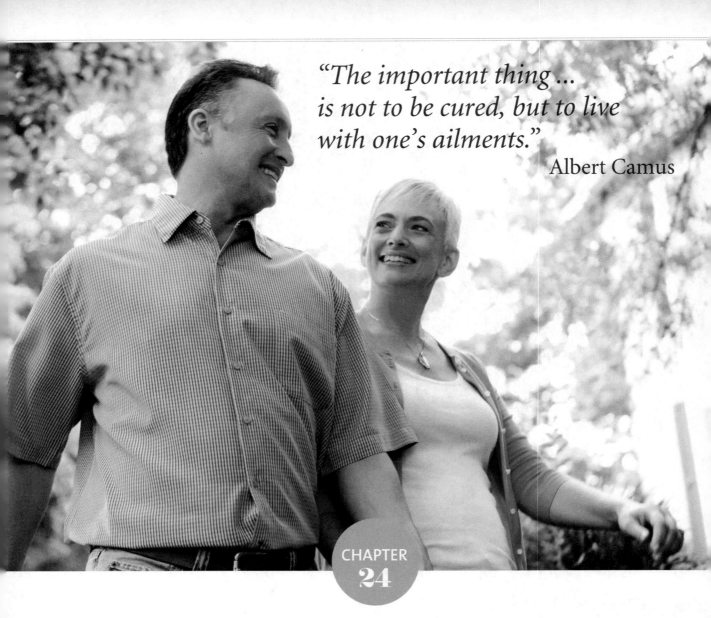

*"The important thing ...
is not to be cured, but to live
with one's ailments."*

Albert Camus

Living Better
with Diabetes

Chapters 24, 25 and 26 address three important psychological challenges related to diabetes: adaptation, stress management, and motivation to change lifestyles. This chapter begins by exploring the mental distress experienced by people with diabetes. It goes on to outline the process of active acceptance by which people with diabetes can integrate the disease and its treatment into their lives. It will also describe certain psychological symptoms – for example, depression, anxiety, and eating disorders – that can arise, potentially complicating adaptation to the disease. A few approaches to these issues are presented, in the hopes of providing some guidance and support to people making the changes required to live – and to live better – with diabetes.

How does diabetes affect a person's daily life?

"Let our despair be the very source of our courage." Seneca

Surprisingly, despite the daily demands of diabetes self-management, some people claim that the disease is the best thing that ever happened to them. Some go so far as to say that they are healthier now, since the diagnosis, while others maintain that diabetes has helped them improve their lifestyles. If you are newly diagnosed with the disease or have been struggling with it for a number of years, these might be astonishing statements. How can diabetes, a chronic disease with serious medical consequences, promote well-being and improve quality of life? How is it that some people with diabetes are able to benefit from their disease, both physically and psychologically?

Before arriving at a realistic view of diabetes and diabetes self-management, people diagnosed with the disease must overcome obstacles, meet challenges, and very likely struggle with feelings of anger, despair, and sadness. Indeed, experiencing this range of emotions is an important stage and can lead to a better psychological adjustment to the disease.

Recent research in the areas of endocrinology, psychiatry, psychology, and nursing care have shown that people that have diabetes are more likely to experience mental distress than people who do not.[17, 3] These studies have provided a deeper insight into what is known as "diabetes-related emotional distress," a concept described by researcher William Polonsky and his team.[12] A frequent topic of study over the last decade, diabetes-related emotional distress has been shown to be even more closely associated than depression with poor blood glucose control.[6, 7, 3] It can also appear alongside depression or lead to it.[19, 9, 11, 20] This type of emotional distress should be recognized and assessed regularly to limit its potentially negative effects on physical and mental health and to promote the person's long-term, optimal adaptation to diabetes and its treatment.[3]

What is diabetes-related emotional distress?

"Courage isn't the absence of fear; it's being able to dominate your fear."
François Mitterrand

Diabetes-related emotional distress can be different in different people. Generally, it involves emotional distress experienced by the person with diabetes upon diagnosis and on a daily basis thereafter when faced with the burdens of diabetes self-care. Here are a few examples from the Problem Areas in Diabetes (PAID) questionnaire[21] of issues relating to diabetes that contribute to emotional distress in people living with the disease who are required to commit to long-term self-care.

- difficulty accepting diabetes and its treatment
- fear, worry, anxiety, anger, despair, and depression when thinking about living with diabetes
- worry about hypoglycemia or hyperglycemia
- feeling discouraged with the treatment plan (blood glucose tests, oral antidiabetic medications, insulin injections, etc.)
- constant concern, loss of pleasure and freedom, or frustration with food, meals, and nutrition requirements
- feelings of guilt or anxiety when diabetes is not fully controlled
- feelings of being overwhelmed by treatment or of not having clear or concrete goals

- feeling burned out by the constant effort needed to manage diabetes
- not knowing if moods or feelings are related to variations in blood glucose levels
- uncomfortable social situations related to diabetes care
- feeling that friends and/or family members are not supportive of diabetes management efforts; feeling alone with the diabetes
- feeling unsatisfied with relationships with doctors (GP, diabetes specialists, ophthalmologists, etc.) and other health professionals (nurses, dietitians, pharmacists, psychologists, etc.)
- worrying about the present, the future, and the possibility of serious complications.

The vigilance required for diabetes self-care exerts daily psychological pressure and forces you to delve deep into your personal tool kit. Living with diabetes requires the management of your energy and resources over the long term, to ensure that your self-care is given the attention it needs. Priorities must be re-evaluated to cope with any diabetes-related emotional distress and prevent diabetes burnout[14] or even the development of serious mental health issues such as depression, anxiety, or eating disorders. Your attitude can also help you deal with the constant pressure it exerts on your life. Try framing it in the following way, for example:

"Since I have to live with diabetes and it causes me a certain amount of distress every day, I should pay particular attention to taking care of myself psychologically and to having fun in a healthy way. This will help me sustain my efforts as I adapt to the disease and ensure that I will have the highest quality of life for the longest time possible."

What are the possible psychological reactions to a diabetes diagnosis?

"What is courage? Nothing but keeping a serene mind and a free spirit in the face of danger." Paul Cazin

When people receive a diagnosis, they usually undergo an emotional shock, although they meay not be fully aware of it. This emotional shock is created by the need to face the reality that the disease will inevitably cause some losses. When the diagnosis is diabetes, whether type 1 or type 2, the perceived or anticipated losses are numerous and varied: loss of health, pleasure, freedom, spontaneity, personal power, autonomy, belonging, and personal efficiency, to name but a few. You may feel as though you can no longer embody certain values that have given your life meaning up until now.

This emotional shock will trigger a grieving process similar to what is experienced when losing a loved one or a job. In other words, your first task is to grieve the loss of your life as it was before diabetes. Life will never be the same, and you will also have to change. Sooner or later, the grieving process will lead to the active acceptance of the diagnosis and then of the requirements of treatment. You must spend a certain amount of time – on average, at least one year after diagnosis – experiencing these intense emotions and rethinking your values and lifestyle so that you can eventually integrate diabetes as harmoniously as possible into your life. In this way, you will come to accept who you used to be, who you are now, and who you hope to become.

This grieving process takes place over a number of stages, corresponding to the different emotions, varying in intensity and duration, that arise in people with diabetes in these circumstances. These emotions are completely normal and, through your daily efforts, will help you evolve towards a new emotional balance and acceptance.

What are the stages leading to an active acceptance of diabetes?

The table on the next page outlines the five stages of grief. Different people can experience the stages in a different order, more quickly or more slowly, more or less consciously, or more or less intensely. Some stages can return, triggered by a change in treatment or the appearance of complications. For example, feelings of injustice and the related anger may return if the doctor proposes a new drug treatment (oral antidiabetic drug, the introduction of insulin therapy, the transition to an insulin pump) or even if the nutrition plan needs adjusting. Some people can become overwhelmed with sadness or despair because of the development of complications such as neuropathic pain or vision loss.

STAGES LEADING TO THE ACTIVE ACCEPTANCE OF CHRONIC ILLNESS

Stage	Description	Characteristic statements
Denial	• Ignoring or trivializing the unbearable aspects of the disease or treatment • Refusing to acknowledge the disease or its seriousness • Completely or partially denying the disease.	• "I don't feel sick, so I can't be diabetic." • "Don't worry, my blood sugar is just a little high." • "I'm not diabetic, I'm borderline diabetic." • "It's okay if I don't test my blood glucose regularly."
Anger	• Seeing the disease as an injustice • Resenting others • Blaming others • Seeing only the negative aspects of treatment	• "Diabetes is the worst disease. It's ruining my life." • "Why is this happening to me?" • "None of my brothers or sisters have it. I'm angry at my parents for giving it to me." • "My doctor didn't tell me clearly that I had diabetes. He should have referred me to a dietitian earlier."
Bargaining	• Acknowledging what is acceptable and ignoring what is not • Acceptance is very conditional	• "I'm taking pills to lower my blood sugar, so I don't need to watch what I eat." • "I take insulin except when I have a business lunch." • "I'm on the pump so I don't have to use a pen injector anymore. But I refuse to test my blood glucose six times a day."
Reflection, resignation, or depression	• Realizing that denying the illness is pointless • Exaggerated perception of limitations • Possible feelings of helplessness or becoming dependant on others	• "No matter what I do, the disease won't go away." • "No matter how much I want to, I can never take a vacation from diabetes." • "Is there any point in living a life like this?" • "I feel like I will never be the same person again." • "I am afraid of being a burden on others."
Acceptance	• Perceiving the disease and its treatment realistically • Taking concrete and positive action acknowledging the reality of the disease and its treatment	• "I would rather not have diabetes, but I don't have a choice so I have to do my best." • "Even though I have diabetes, I am healthy. I exercise more and eat better than I did before."

How is the grieving process resolved and acceptance achieved?

"There is only one reality: to live.
But there are a thousand ways to do it."
Gilbert Choquette.

Managing your emotions through the grieving process is the first difficult and necessary stage. Becoming aware of how your emotions are affecting your body can help you put a name to them (emotions related to anxiety, hostility, guilt, shame, or sadness) and identify the automatic thoughts triggering them. The table on the next page shows the emotions that can be associated with the stages of the grieving process and some possible triggering thoughts. The table can help you identify your emotions more clearly, bringing you closer to a nonjudgmental acceptance of your emotions, which is an essential element of the healthy management of your emotional and psychological states. Indeed, living with diabetes is not easy. Although the disease is increasingly common, its impact is too often trivialized or exaggerated. Accepting your emotions openly is your way of acknowledging your right to feel them and allowing them to simply exist.

Finally, it is important to express your emotions in whatever way works for you, whether in writing, in song, or through visual art. A healthy expression of emotions is encouraged. Suppressing them or preventing yourself from expressing them – for example, tamping them down and hiding them from others, putting up a brave face – requires a lot of focus and energy. Moreover, it will not reduce the intensity of your feelings.[16, 10] If you express what you are feeling clearly and in a healthy way, your emotions will be less intense and it will require less effort to deal with them. You can then be a bit more open, a bit more available to others – in a way, free of the weight of your emotions. This will give you the energy to adapt to your diabetes – that is, to understand the recommendations about self-care and to face the inevitable daily changes it brings.

FAMILIES OF EMOTIONS AND THE AUTOMATIC THOUGHTS THAT TRIGGER THEM, ADAPTED TO THE CONTEXT OF DIABETES

Families of emotions	Examples of automatic thoughts triggering these emotions
ANXIETY Dread, worry, fear, apprehension, doubt, stress, panic, concern	• "Diabetes is a threat to my health. I can't avoid the risks of complications." • "I can't decide whether or not to be diabetic. My only power is to deny that I have it." • "Diabetes caused someone I love to die."
HOSTILITY Impatience, irritation, anger, rage, hatred, disgust, desire for vengeance, aggressiveness	• "Diabetes happened because someone failed to tell me in time that I was at risk." • "Diabetes should not be part of my life. I don't deserve it."
GUILT, LOW SELF-ESTEEM, SHAME Regret, remorse, self-blame, feeling of impotence, mistrust	• "Diabetes is my own fault. I didn't take care of myself." • "I shouldn't have put off seeing the doctor. I take care of everyone else, so I should have known how to prevent what is happening to me." • "My colleagues won't see me the same way if they learn that I have diabetes."
SADNESS Disappointment, dejection, discouragement, despair	• "I can't go back and change the course of events. I have been diagnosed with diabetes." • "I have a chronic disease, which means I have to live with it forever. I'll never make it."
JOY, LOVE, PRIDE	• "The diabetes treatment is good for me." • "I was able to express my needs to my doctor, and he helped me prevent my hypoglycemia." • "I have been able to do more exercise! I can do this." • "I know how to count carbohydrates, and I take care of myself by injecting the corresponding amount of insulin."

Adapted from the table in Chaloult, L. (2008) *La thérapie cognitivo-comportementale : Théorie et pratique*, page 190. Montreal: Gaëtan Morin.

Is it true that people with diabetes change personalities and become angry or aggressive?

No. Anger is not a personality trait of people with diabetes. There may be people with diabetes whose personalities are angry, but this has nothing to do with their diabetes.

Anger is an emotion in the hostility family (*see table on page 227*) that anyone can experience, but is also part of the normal process of active acceptance of a chronic disease. It is not unique to people with diabetes; anyone with a chronic disease who is struggling to accept it will feel it. Irritability can simply be the **manifestation of a person's difficulty in actively accepting the disease.**

Emotions such as irritability and anger are properly understood as signals that one of **your needs, which you perceive as important, are not being fulfilled either partially or completely** in a situation involving diabetes. The recommended approach is to **specifically identify** the emotion and to accept it so that you can express it in a healthy way – in other words, by making a clear, verbal statement asserting your personal experience. Anger can give you the energy to find constructive ways to have your needs and values met, while remaining aware of the demands of both the chronic illness and the people around you.

However, **a sudden change of personality or mood revealing itself as irritability or anger could be a sign of hypoglycemia.** If so, the signs will disappear as soon as blood glucose is corrected. In this case, anger or irritability is a signal of a physiological need to provide your body and brain with more energy. The correct approach is to take a blood glucose reading and proceed with the recommended treatment to correct the hypoglycemia.

Mood changes can also occur when you become **very tired** because your blood sugar levels are very high (**hyperglycemia**) or fluctuating (varying rapidly from hyperglycemia to hypoglycemia or vice-versa). These mood changes usually stop rather quickly once blood glucose levels are controlled and energy returns.

It is important that your family, friends, and co-workers understand the reasons for your mood changes and provide help when required. An environment of acceptance and mutual respect can make it easier to regulate feelings of anger or irritability.

How do I achieve the final stage of active acceptance?

"It often requires more courage to change your opinions than to hold true to them."
Friedrich Hebbel

To promote the healthy management of emotions and, ultimately, to be as realistic and positive as possible about the disease, you may have to change some of your **beliefs** and **behaviours**.

The process of change is made easier by a **better understanding of diabetes**. Remain informed by reading books (like this one), taking part in information workshops, and speaking with your doctor or a health professional. A number of myths about diabetes still exist, and they can cause initial reactions that either trivialize the disease or exaggerate the dangers. They may cause you to focus only on the bad aspects and prevent you from looking for the resources and means that are available to help you adapt.

Up-to-date information about diabetes will debunk myths and **modify your belief systems** and attitudes about the disease and self-care. Your new knowledge will lead you to **change your behaviour and make the right treatment choices in collaboration with your doctor and diabetes care team**. Adapting your thoughts and behaviours can calm some of your fears and soothe your frustration, while also making you feel less powerless in the face of the disease.

Long-term active acceptance involves a **daily effort to remain motivated to perform actions with positive consequences** on your blood glucose. Ultimately, the benefits of your efforts will inspire a sense of pride and confidence.

Finally, adjusting your beliefs and your behaviours to the reality of diabetes and its treatment will **improve your emotions**, quality of life, and energy levels, and have a positive effect on your present and future psychological well-being.

Is there any good news for a person who has just been diagnosed with diabetes?

In the first year following diagnosis, you might find it hard to believe that your treatment will help your moods, give you more energy in the short term, and prevent complications in the medium and long term. The more you learn about recent scientific advances in the area of diabetes, however the more reasons you will have to be optimistic. Indeed, based on the recent *Clinical Practice Guidelines* of the Canadian Diabetes Association,[3] which is supported by recent research, you have every right to be hopeful and to believe that:

- diabetes **can be well controlled**;
- good blood glucose control considerably reduces the risk of serious long-term complications long-term;
- information and training resources such as individual or group diabetes education programs are effective ways of acquiring the skills needed to **adapt your diabetes**

treatment to the changing circumstances of your everyday life and individual needs;

- diabetes is an opportunity to learn how to eat better, exercise regularly, more effectively manage stress, regulate your emotions, and improve your quality of life – in short, to live better.

As you live with diabetes on a daily basis, you will experience the benefits of treatment and gain the confidence needed to make changes while maintaining control over your blood glucose levels and your disease in general. Self-awareness, tolerance and perseverance are crucial traits that make it possible to enjoy a long, active, healthy and satisfying life.

How can the process of actively accepting diabetes be described briefly?

You may never be happy that you have diabetes. Nevertheless, you can still integrate the demands of the disease and its treatment into your life as harmoniously as possible. Once you see yourself performing the daily actions required to manage and treat diabetes, while taking into account your own personal needs and values, then you will know that you have accepted your diabetes.

The process of accepting diabetes requires:
- managing your emotions in a healthy way;
- re-examining your beliefs and perceptions of the disease and its treatment, and adjusting them as needed to be more realistic;
- reorganizing your priorities and personal values, if necessary;
- learning through your self-care experiences that your treatment is beneficial to you;
- realizing that you can overcome the obstacles to treatment and resolve the issues it raises, thereby developing a sense of competence with respect to your diabetes;
- remaining informed on current developments in the area of diabetes and putting your knowledge into action by focusing on your health through your commitment to self-care;
- maintaining your quality of life as much as possible by meeting your needs and upholding your personal values, while taking your diabetes into account on a daily basis.

There are tools available to support you as you move towards an active acceptance of your diabetes. For example, in 2008 Diabetes Quebec published a guide (in French) that was recognized as the best educational material published by that organization that year. It contains practical exercises to help you orient yourself in your process that urge you to re-examine some of your beliefs about diabetes and to boost your confidence to make changes. Although written for people with type 2 diabetes, the exercises are also useful for people with type 1.

This book can be ordered from Diabetes Quebec by mail, fax or online at

- http://www.diabete.qc.ca/html/materiel_publications/prod_edu.html#suivez
- Lapointe, J. (2008). *Accepter son diabète : suivez le guide. À l'intention des personnes diabétiques de type 2 pour les aider à accepter et à prendre en charge leur diabète.* Diabetes Quebec, 24 pages.

Are there specific types of emotional distress that are common among people with diabetes?

Yes. Studies have suggested that depression, anxiety disorders, and eating disorders (anorexia, bulimia, and binge eating), while quite common in general population, are even more prevalent in people with diabetes.[3]

It is estimated that depression is up to three times more frequent in people with diabetes than in the general population. According to the *Clinical Practice Guidelines* of the Canadian Diabetes Association,[3] approximately 30% of people with diabetes have symptoms of depression and 10% have major depression (double the incidence in people without a chronic disease). Some studies have shown that up to 25% of people with diabetes experience depression.[8]

Similarly, anxiety issues are more frequent in people with diabetes. A study cited by the Canadian Diabetes Association[3] demonstrates that 14% of people with diabetes also suffer from generalized anxiety disorder (nearly three times more than the general population). Symptoms of anxiety are up to three times more frequent in people with diabetes (ranging from 30% to 40%). Anxiety is frequently experienced simultaneously with depression.

Eating disorders (anorexia, bulimia, binge eating) are more frequent in people with type 1 and type 2 diabetes than in people in the general population.[3] People with diabetes are often concerned about their weight and nutrition, and can sometimes feel as though they are "feeding their feelings." One study has shown that people with diabetes are more likely to engage in compulsive overeating or binge eating to soothe their emotional distress.[5] Compulsive overeating may also be related to an increase in blood glucose control issues, physical inactivity, and obesity. Moreover, people with binge eating disorder are significantly more likely than people who do not suffer from it to experience depression (between 60% and 70% of cases) and anxiety (30% to 50% of cases). According to the Canadian Diabetes Association,[3] an average of 50% of people with diabetes also have symptoms of depression and one eating disorder (anorexia, bulimia, or binge eating).

It is very important to diagnose depression, anxiety, and eating disorders in people with diabetes. These issues can weaken the motivation needed for self-management and as a result have negative consequences on their blood glucose control.

How is depression recognized?

First, it is important to understand the difference between sadness, which is a normal emotion that plays a part in the grieving process, and major depression, which is a mental health issue. A person who feels sad will not necessarily be diagnosed with depression.

Depression is diagnosed when the following symptoms have lasted at least two weeks and have begun affecting your work and social life:
- feeling low, sad, hopeless, discouraged, "unable to go on," practically all day, every day;
- loss of interest or pleasure in almost all activities;
- unexplained loss of appetite or weight loss or significant increase in appetite and weight gain;
- insomnia or a need to sleep more than usual;
- agitation (e.g., difficulty sitting still) or the slowing down of psychomotor functions (e.g., slowed speech, monotone voice, slow to answer questions, slower bodily movements);
- lack of energy, tiredness;
- feelings of loss of dignity, self-blame, excessive or inappropriate guilt;
- difficulty concentrating, thinking, or making a decision;
- morbid thoughts or thoughts of death, suicidal ideation, death wishes, or suicide attempts.

What should I do if I think I am suffering from depression?

If you feel some or several of these symptoms for at least two weeks, tell your doctor. He or she will determine if they are due to diabetes, another physical problem (e.g., hypothyroidism), or depression. Your doctor can then recommend the appropriate treatment or refer you to a mental health specialist, if appropriate.

Although sadness is often a normal part of the grieving process after a diabetes diagnosis, it is important to see a doctor if it intensifies and last several weeks.

Depression is one of the easiest mental health issues to treat, especially if diagnosed early. Most people are prescribed antidepressant drugs and/or cognitive-behavioural therapy. The combination of these two approaches has been recognized as the most efficient and is recommended by the Canadian Diabetes Association.[3] The support of your family, friends, and support groups (e.g., Revivre, Groupe d'Entraide G.E.M.E.) are also important.

How are anxiety disorders recognized?

Anxiety disorders are mental health problems in which anxiety is the predominant disturbance. In people with diabetes, anxiety disorders such as phobias (e.g., fear of needles, fear of low blood glucose) and generalized anxiety are the most frequent.

Generalized anxiety disorder may be diagnosed if you have the following symptoms:
- anxiety and excessive worry most of the time, for at least six months, about different events or activities;
- difficulty controlling these worries;
- intense distress;
- agitation, feeling on edge;
- easily fatigued;
- difficulty concentrating or memory lapses;
- irritability;
- muscle tension;
- disturbed sleep.

What should I do if I think I am suffering from an anxiety disorder?

If you are showing signs of an anxiety disorder, speak to your doctor, who will evaluate your situation, recommend the appropriate treatment, and refer you to a mental health professional, if appropriate.

Anxiety disorders can be treated with drugs and/or psychotherapy. Common therapeutic tools include relaxation techniques such as abdominal breathing and meditation. Support groups (e.g., **Phobies-Zéro** or **La Clé des Champs**) and the encouragement of your friends and family are also excellent and helpful resources.

How is binge eating (compulsive overeating) recognized?

Binge eating (also referred to as compulsive overeating) is considered to be an eating disorder distinct from bulimia and anorexia.[2] According to the fifth edition of the *Diagnostic and Statistical Manual of Mental Disorders* (DSM-V) published in May of 2013, a person is diagnosed with **binge eating disorder** when the following behaviour is observed:

1 Eating an abnormal amount of food within a given period of time, combined with a feeling of a loss of control during this period; the person is unable to control the amount of food ingested and cannot stop eating.

2 Experiencing three of the following five states:
   - eating more quickly than usual;
   - eating until uncomfortably full;
   - eating large amounts of food even when not hungry;
   - eating alone because of embarrassment and shame about how much the person is eating;
   - feeling disgusted, depressed, or guilty after a binge.

The person also feels very distressed about the binges. Binge overeating happens at least twice a week for at least six months, and the person does not compensate for the behaviour (e.g., by inducing vomiting, exercising more intensely, or taking laxatives). The binges may also take place only at night (night eating syndrome).

What should I do if I think I am suffering from binge eating disorder?

Speak to your doctor or another health professional who can direct you to the appropriate resources (e.g., psychologist, psychotherapist, and/or dietitian) for treatment. As someone with diabetes, you should see your doctor even if the binges are less frequent than what is necessary for a medical diagnosis, since it is recognized that binge eating by a person with diabetes, even when infrequent, increases the risk of complications, hampers adhesion to the treatment plan, and is not conducive to blood glucose control.[1]

Treatment for binge eating includes education, nutritional intervention, psychotherapy, and/or drugs. Since obesity is frequently associated with binge eating, the person should receive information about this issue as well. In terms of the nutrition plan, the most effective approach is one that promotes moderation – and not restriction – both at meals and in between,[15, 18] since periods of deprivation can actually trigger a binge. Tools enabling the healthy management of emotions associated with the disorder (e.g., shame, anxiety, anger, powerlessness, and self-criticism) are often used. It is important to remember that the effective treatment of binge eating generally does not lead to weight loss, although it does promote better control over the diabetes and a better sense of psychological well-being – two things that are needed before undertaking a weight-loss diet.

Anorexia and Bulimia Quebec has a helpline and can provide references and services for people with anorexia, bulimia, or binge eating disorder.

Where can I find resources to help me if I have diabetes and I am suffering from emotional distress?

First, talk to your doctor. In some cases, drug treatment can be indicated. Alternatively, your doctor might refer you to a mental health specialist (psychiatrist, psychologist, or psychotherapist) with a public practice or to another health professional (nurse, dietitian, pharmacist, or kinesiologist), who can meet your specific needs and provide you with support.

If you wish to consult a mental health specialist directly, information is available through most CLSCs (community service centres) and CSSSs (health and social services centres). Your doctor could also refer you to the psychology department or psychiatric unit of a hospital.

A psychologist or psychotherapist specializing in diabetes and working in private practice is another option. Contact information can be obtained through the Ordre des Psychologues du Québec (Quebec order of psychologists; *see chapter 28, "Resources"*).

Remember

The way you manage your diabetes is influenced by your personality, experience, values, and beliefs.

You cannot control how long the grieving process will take, but you can do your best to manage your emotions about diabetes in a healthy way.

Actively informing yourself about diabetes will give you the opportunity to re-examine your perspective on the disease and learn how to see it more realistically.

When it comes to your diabetes management, you play the lead. Although diabetes is a chronic, incurable disease, you — with the help of your health care team — have the power to control your blood glucose through your every day actions and to prevent or limit the development of complications of diabetes.

As you move forward with diabetes, be sure to take care of your mental health and seek out any support you may need to safeguard your physical health and quality of life.

Bibliography

1 Alloway, S. C., Toth, E. L. & McCargar, L. J. (2001). Effectiveness of a group psychoeducation program for the treatment of subclinical disordered eating in women with type 1 diabetes. *Canadian Journal of Dietetic Practice and Research*, 62(4), 188-92.

2 American Psychiatric Association. (2000). DSM-IV: *Diagnostic and Statistical Manual of Mental Disorders*, 4th ed. American Psychiatric Association.

3 Canadian Diabetes Association Clinical Practice Guidelines Expert Committee. (2013). Canadian Diabetes Association 2013 Clinical Practice Guidelines for the Prevention and Management of Diabetes in Canada: Diabetes and mental health. *Canadian Journal of Diabetes*, 37(suppl 1), S87-S92. Accessed: http://www.guidelines.diabetes.ca.

4 Chaloult, L. (2008). *La thérapie cognitivo-comportementale : Théorie et pratique*. Montreal, QC : Gaëtan Morin.

5 Deboer, L. B., Tart, C. D., Presnell, K. E., Powers, M. B., Baldwin, A. S., & Smits, J. A. (2012). Physical activity as a moderator of the association between anxiety sensitivity and binge eating. E*ating Behaviors*, 13(3), 194-201. Accessed: doi: 10.1016/j.eatbeh.2012.01.009.

6 Fisher, L., Skaff, M. M., Mullan, J. T., Arean, P., Mohr, D., Masharan, U., Glasgow, R., & Laurencin, G. (2007). Clinical depression versus distress among patients with type 2 diabetes: not just a question of semantics. *Diabetes Care*, 30(3), 542-548.

7 Fisher L., Mullan, J. T., Arean, P., Glasgow, R. E., Hessler, D., & Masharani U. (2010). Diabetes distress but not clinical depression or depressive symptoms is associated with glycemic control in both cross-sectional and longitudinal analyses. *Diabetes Care*, 33(1), 23-28.

8 Fisher, E. B., Chan, J. C., Nan, H., Sartorius, N., & Oldenburg, B. F. (2012). Co-occurrence of diabetes and depression: conceptual considerations for an emerging global health challenge. J*ournal of Affective Disorders*, 142, s56-s66.

9 Gois C., Akiskal H., Akiskal K., & Figueira, M. L. (2012). Depressive temperament, distress, psychological adjustment and depressive symptoms in type 2 diabetes. *Journal of Affective Disorders*, 143(1-3), 1-4. Accessed: doi:10.1016/j.jad.2012.05.028.

10 Krauth-Gruber, S. (2009). La régulation des émotions. *Revue électronique de Psychologie Sociale*, 4, 32-39.

11 Lloyd, C., Pouwer, F., & Hermanns, N. (2012). S*creening for Depression and other Psychological problems in Diabetes*. London: Springer.

12 Polonsky, Anderson, Lohrer, Welch, Jacobson, Aponte & Schwartz, 1995

13 Polonsky, W. H., Anderson, B. J., Lohrer, P. A., Welch, G., Jacobson, A. M., Aponte, J. E., & Schwartz, C. E. (1995). Assessment of diabetes-related distress. *Diabetes Care*, 18, 754-60.

14 Polonsky W. H. (1999). Diabetes Burnout: *What to Do When You Can't Take It Anymore*. Alexandria, Virginia: American Diabetes Association.

15 Racine, S. E., Culbert, K. M., Larson, C. L., & Klump, K. L. (2009). The moderating effects of impulsivity and dietary restraint on associations between serotonin genes and binge eating. *Journal of Psychiatric Research*, 43, 1278-1286.

16 Richards, J. M., & Gross, J. J. (1999). Composure at any cost? The cognitive consequences of emotion suppression. *Personality and Social Psychology Bulletin*, 25, 1033-1044.

17 Shin, J. K., Chiu, Y. L., Choi, S., Cho, S., Bang, H. (2012). Serious psychological distress, health risk behaviors, and diabetes care among adults with type 2 diabetes: the California Health Interview Survey 2007. *Diabetes Research and Clinical Practice*, 95(3), 406-14. Accessed: doi:10.1016/j.diabres.2011.10.043.

18 Stotland, S., & Beauchemin, A. (2011). Restraint, moderation and the stages of weight self-regulation: Implications for CBT for obesity. *Canadian Journal of Diabetes*, 35(2), 154.

19 Sullivan, Evans, Anderson, O'Connor, Raisch, Simmons, Narayan, ACCORD Trial, 2012.

20 Sullivan, M. D., Evans, G., Anderson, R., O'Connor, P., Raisch, D. W., Simmons, D. L. & Narayan, V. K. M. (2012). Diabetes Symptoms and Distress in ACCORD Trial Participants: Relationship to Baseline Clinical Variables. *Clinical Diabetes*, 30, 101-108. Accessed: doi:10.2337/diaclin.30.3.101.

21 Sultan S, Heurtier-Hartemann A. (2001). Coping and distress as predictors of glycemic control in diabetes. *Journal of Health Psychology*, 6, 731-739.

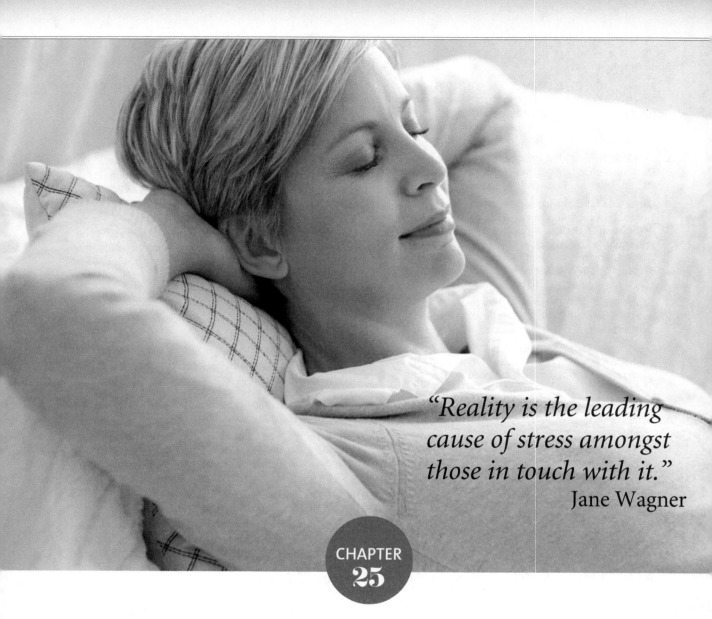

"*Reality is the leading cause of stress amongst those in touch with it.*"
Jane Wagner

Managing Daily Stress

Because diabetes and its treatment are potential sources of mental distress, it is all the more important for people with the disease to learn how to manage stress in their everyday lives. This chapter will identify potential stressors and their possible effects, while listing various ways of dealing with them. While it might be impossible to eliminate stress from our modern lives, it is within our power to recognize its sources, adapt our reactions accordingly and, when circumstances permit, resolve the problems or obtain the support we need to face them better. Relaxation and pleasure may be a bit more challenging for people with diabetes, but it is far from impossible.

What is stress?

Life is stressful because of the constant need to react and adapt to changes taking place both inside and around us. Most of the time, these demands are not overwhelming; however, as Dr. Hans Selye, endocrinologist and originator of the concept, points out, stress is always with us (Selye, 1936).

The term "stress" is often used informally to refer to stressful situations or sources of stress, both of which should properly be referred to as "stressors." The most common type of "**stress**," which is also the subject of this chapter, is **the physical or psychological feeling experienced when we are in a situation that we perceive to be threatening and beyond our capacity to deal with effectively.** These are situations in which most people feel "stressed." A stressful situation generally has four characteristics: it is perceived to be uncontrollable, unpredictable, unfamiliar, and threatening to the ego. The brain triggers an adaptation reaction in the body that is based on the perception of the event, not merely the event itself.

Why should a person with diabetes be concerned about everyday stress?

For people with diabetes, the effects of stress are apparent and harmful because stress can **increase blood glucose levels**. If your blood glucose readings reveal hyperglycemia, it may be at least in part explained by a stressful situation you are experiencing. Stress acts directly on blood glucose by stimulating the secretion of **stress hormones** – adrenaline, ACTH (adrenocorticotropic hormone), cortisol, oxytocin, and vasopressin – that release glucose reserves in the liver into the blood, decreasing the effect of insulin by increasing resistance to it in the cells.

Stress can also act **indirectly** by affecting **behaviour**, causing people to be less vigilant about their self-care. Some people under stress might, for example, find themselves snacking more frequently, doing less exercise, or forgetting to take their medication, contributing to an increase in blood glucose levels. In principle, once the stressful situation has passed, blood glucose returns to normal on its own within a day. If the stress is chronic and ongoing, however – for example, after losing a loved one or a job – blood glucose can remain higher than usual for anywhere from a few days to several months.

Other people react to stress by losing their appetite, skipping meals, sleeping less, or becoming hyperactive (e.g., finding themselves doing housework more vigorously, getting caught in spiralling thoughts, or skipping breaks at work). In these cases, stress can lead indirectly to isolated hypoglycemic episodes, which should be corrected by following a doctor's recommendations. This indirect effect can be prevented by maintaining stable eating and sleeping habits and by avoiding hyperactivity when faced with a stressor.

Does stress cause diabetes?
No. It might be a trigger, however, in people who are genetically predisposed. It is also generally agreed that stress can complicate blood glucose self-management, thereby contributing to the appearance of complications of diabetes.

What is the difference between "good" stress and "bad" stress?
Everyone has a different resistance to stress. Therefore, depending on a number of factors, stress can be experienced as either good or bad, either a challenge or a crushing burden.

What really determines whether stress is perceived to be good or bad is our individual capacity to deal with a threatening situation – in other words, our "**feeling of personal effectiveness**" with respect to diabetes. Stress can be a positive force: you may find, for example, that solving a difficult problem or falling in love causes good stress because it increases pleasure and satisfaction in your life. If you believe that you do not have the capacity to deal with events like these, however, they will probably cause you a great deal of stress, which you will experience as "bad."

⑤

What are the sources of stress?

There are several broad categories of stressors in our lives, including:

- physical stressors: disease and its consequences, fatigue, pain;
- psychological stressors: emotions, attitudes, behaviours;
- social stressors: interpersonal and professional relationships, the death of a loved one, life changes (e.g., marriage, moving, retirement).

If you have diabetes, whatever the intensity of the **physical stressors** you are experiencing – be it the flu, cancer, or anything in between – you are likely to see an increase in your blood glucose because your body is fighting the disease. Fatigue and pain also cause stress reactions in the body. The following books can help you better understand the mechanisms involved in the management of diabetes, fatigue, and pain, and find some solutions to limit their impact on your stress levels:

- Gauthier, M. (2010). *Fatigue chronique : causes, symptômes, traitements.* Montreal: Les Éditions Option Santé.
- Rivard, M.-J. & Gringras, D. (2012). *La douleur: de la souffrance au mieux-être.* Montreal: Trécarré.
- Savard, J. (2010). *Faire face au cancer – avec la pensée réaliste.* Quebec City: Flammarion Québec.

When the situation involves **psychological stressors** such as depression or anxiety, it is often a good idea to reflect on the issues and make an effort to manage your emotions, adjust your attitudes, and modify your behaviours. Here are some books that can help:

- Addis, M. E. & Martell, C. R. (2004). *Overcoming Depression One Step at a Time: The New Behavioural Activation Approach to Getting Your Life Back.* New York: New Harbinger Press.
- André, C. & Muz (2002). *Petites angoisses et grosses phobies.* Paris: Éditions du Seuil.
- Ladouceur, R., Bélanger, L. & Léger, E. (2003). *Arrêter de vous faire du souci pour tout et pour rien.* Paris: Éditions Odile Jacob.
- Marchand, A. & Letarte, A. (2004). *La peur d'avoir peur.* Montreal: Éditions Stanké.
- Trickett, S. (2003). *Libérez-vous : comment vous débarrasser de l'anxiété et de la dépression* Montreal: Éditions Caractère.
- Willard, M. (2012) *La dépression au travail: prévenir et surmonter.* Paris: Éditions Odile Jacob.
- Young, J. E. (2003) *Je réinvente ma vie.* Montreal: Les Éditions de l'Homme.

Social stressors caused by your relationships with other people, professional lives, and life events are also significant opportunities for reflection and change. Happy events (marriage, the birth of a child, a promotion) and difficult events (separation, loss of a job, death of a loved one) are both potential sources of stress. Here are a few more reading suggestions:

- Brillon, P. (2012). *Quand la mort est traumatique*. Montreal: Les Éditions Québécor.
- Halpern, H. (2013). *Choisir qui on aime: de la dépendance à l'autonomie*. Montreal: Les Éditions de l'Homme.
- Lelord, F. & André, C. (2000). *Comment gérer les personnalités difficiles*. Paris: Éditions du Seuil.
- Michaud, I. (2012) *Guide pour mieux faire face à une perte d'emploi*. Montreal: Les Éditions Québécor.
- Monbourquette, J. (2004). *Grandir : aimer, perdre et grandir*. Montreal: Les Éditions Novalis.

What influences our resistance to stress?

Not only does resistance to stress vary from person to person, it also fluctuates within the same person, depending on the specific challenges and time of life. Your resistance to stress is influenced by **personal factors** such as your temperament, personality, genetics, past experiences, and attitudes. The emotions you feel – guilt, anxiety, sadness, fear, anger, etc. – and the way you manage them will affect whether stress is easy or difficult for you to face. Mobilizing your **personal resources** – by adopting adaptation strategies (problem solving, relaxation techniques, etc.) and seeking out support or information, for example – can also help you better cope with the stressors in your life.

How do I recognize the symptoms of stress?

The glucometer exists to check blood glucose levels, but unfortunately, the "stressometer" has yet to be invented. Stress can be difficult to recognize. Some people feel it right away, while others can endure it for long periods without being aware that they have been internalizing stress that is potentially harmful. It is important for you to understand how you react to stress and what symptoms you are likely to show; the table below presents a list of possible symptoms that can help you identify your reactions.

While it is possible to adequately deal with occasional stress, when it is long-lasting, intense, and frequent, it can wear down the body and have undesirable physical consequences. Stress is part of life. Although it can never be eliminated, it can be managed and its negative effects minimized.

PHYSICAL, PSYCHOLOGICAL AND BEHAVIOURAL SYMPTOMS IN THE PRESENCE OF STRESSOR(S)		
Physical symptoms	Psychological symptoms	Behavioural symptoms
• increased heart rate • ncreased blood pressure • increased muscle tension • increased breathing rate • chronic fatigue • headache, backache • chest tightness • digestion problems • loss of appetite	• aggression • irritability • depression • crying jags • inability to cry • feeling drained • feeling dissatisfied • ambivalence • lowered motivation • lowered self-esteem • nightmares • decrease in concentration and attention • forgetting • indecisiveness	• tics • explosions of anger • hypercritical attitude • reduced productivity • increased consumption of certain foods • increased substance consumption (tobacco, alcohol, medications) • sleeping problems • sexual issues

What are three simple steps to help me deal with stress?

1 **Recognize that you are stressed:** First, recognize your individual symptoms. Becoming aware of how you feel is a necessary and useful starting point.

2 **Identify the source:** Identify sources of positive stress, which you perceive as challenges you feel equipped to face, and negative stress, which you experience as overwhelming.

3 **Develop techniques to help you adapt:** When faced with so-called negative stress, develop a personalized plan to reinforce your resistance and deal with the stress as effectively as possible. Research suggests that better results are obtained when people apply a problem-solving technique instead of merely expressing their emotions.

(9)

What are problem-solving techniques?

A person applying a problem-solving technique perceives the stressor as a challenge that requires reflection, analysis, and an exploration of possible solutions. This stage should be followed by action and an evaluation of the outcome. It is quite rare for a problem to be solved in one attempt with no need for adjustment. Unforeseen obstacles or a lack of resources are signs that new solutions are necessary.

SUMMARY OF THE PROBLEM-SOLVING TECHNIQUE

LIST THE PROBLEMS Describe them in concrete terms Begin with the most important	1. 2. 3. 4.		
SET OBJECTIVES Be specific Be realistic Set a time limits	1. 2. 3. 4.		
BRAINSTORM SOLUTIONS; BE CREATIVE AND NON-JUDGMENTAL	1. 2. 3. 4.		
DESCRIBE THE ADVANTAGES AND DISADVANTAGES FOR EACH SOLUTION	Solutions	Disadvantages	Advantages
	1.		
	2.		
	3.		
	4.		
CHOOSE ONE SOLUTION	Solution selected:		
EVALUATE THE OBSTACLES AND THE RESOURCES NEEDED TO IMPLEMENT THE SOLUTION	Obstacles: Resources		
LIST THE STAGES REQUIRED TO IMPLEMENT THE SOLUTION	1. 2. 3. 4. 5.		

Table adapted from Chaloult, L. (2008) *La thérapie cognitivo-comportementale : Théorie et pratique.*[1] Montreal: Gaëtan Morin, appendix 6, pages 16-17.

What are some adaptation techniques that can help me manage everyday stress?

In brief:

- **Manage your emotions:** Learn to identify your negative emotions and express them appropriately to yourself and others. State your own needs, while respecting those of others, and seek out emotional support when needed.

- **Restructure some of your ways of thinking:** Learn how to encourage yourself, avoiding dramatic or self-deprecating thoughts and seeing yourself as a victim. Use positive affirmations to manage paralyzing emotions (e.g., "I can do it," "I've seen worse than this," "That's okay, it's a step in the right direction."). Assess situations as realistically as possible.

- **Change some of your behaviours:** Assert yourself. Give yourself permission to say no when you cannot or do not want to say yes. Do not let problems pile up. Organize your time and set realistic deadlines. Act.

- **Find healthy ways to unwind:** Use relaxation techniques to diminish your stress symptoms. Begin a regular, balanced program of exercise, creative activities, and/or relaxation. Look for activities that are fun and that will expand your horizons, and of course avoid overeating, drinking alcohol, or smoking.

More specifically, people with diabetes who are under stress should check their blood glucose, eat well, exercise, and take medication to treat their diabetes. Maintaining your healthy habits through difficult times will ensure that you keep your blood glucose levels on track. Speak to your doctor immediately about any stress you may be going through, particularly if you observe variations in your blood glucose levels; he or she may suggest a treatment change or refer you to new resources, which can be re-evaluated once the stressful issues have been resolved.

What do relaxation techniques involve?

Relaxation is a useful stress-management tool. Stress produces a number of reactions that activate the body and increase physiological functions (cardiovascular, respiratory, muscular). Relaxation calms them down, re-establishing physiological or psychological balance. Results are more than physical, as relaxation can also have a profound soothing effect on emotions and thoughts. Leisure activities (e.g., exercise, artistic creation, reading) can be just as calming as exercises developed for the sole purpose of relaxation.

Are there any easy relaxation techniques?

There are many. Among the most well-known are active relaxation, which involves alternating tension with relaxation, and passive relaxation, which involves gradual relaxation as you silently guide your awareness from one part of the body to the next. There is also yoga, an ancient Indian practice that is currently very popular, through which physical poses are used to control the functions of the body and seek spiritual enlightenment. In addition, mindfulness meditation encourages practitioners to focus on the sensations apparent to the mind at a given moment, and to observe how they appear, how long they last, and how they disappear. Mindfulness, a practice that derives from Buddhism, has contemporary applications in cognitive psychotherapy as a way to manage stress and treat depression.

Although the relationship between stress and diabetes has long been established in the scientific literature,[3] research on the effectiveness of relaxation techniques for people with the disease is still relatively recent. Some studies on people with diabetes suggest that relaxation techniques (yoga, mindfulness meditation) are potentially beneficial both physiologically (e.g., 0.5% decrease in A1C, improved blood glucose control) and psychologically (e.g., improved quality of life, reduced diabetes-related emotional distress).[2, 4, 5, 6]

Try this simple relaxation technique:
Stop. Remove yourself from external stimuli (noise, light, activity). Sit down, close your eyes, and breathe deeply, finding your own rhythm. After a few minutes, your breathing should slow down. Take an inventory of every part of your body, starting with your feet and ending with your head. You should experience feelings of relaxation, warmth, heaviness, and stillness. With practice, five minutes will be enough time to reach this state. Eventually, you will be able to do it anywhere, even in a public place. This technique is easy, effective, and accessible – all you need is a little practice.

Are there any relaxation tools?

There are a number of recordings on the market, so it is worth trying a few and finding one that works for you. They can be purchased as CDs or downloaded in digital format and loaded onto your iPod or other mp3 player. A portable audio player is a discreet, accessible way of listening to these recordings, whether at work, on public transit, or at home. Many libraries offer a selection; experiment with a few before you make an investment. Here are a few suggestions for beginners:

- Sabourin, M. (1992). *Techniques de relaxation v. 1: relaxation active (technique Jacobson) et relaxation passive (technique suggestive)*. BMG Musique.
- Sabourin, M. (1991). *Techniques de relaxation v. 2 : relaxation autogène (technique de Schultz/Luthe) et imagerie dirigée*. BMG Musique.
- Bordeleau, N. (2006). *Méditation pour mieux vivre (3 CD) : CD 1 Présentation / Méditations guidées; CD 2 Relaxations Guidées; CD 3 Méditations pour Mieux Vivre*. Studio Yogamonde Productions.
- Bordeleau, N. (2004). *Yoga session 1 : Anti-stress*. Studio Yogamonde Productions.
- Kabat-Zin, J. (2005). *Guided Mindfulness Meditation + CD*. Sounds True.
- Kabat-Zin, J. (2007). *Arriving at Your Own Door: 108 Lessons in Mindfulness*. Hyperion.

Relaxation audio recordings are also available online for download, free of charge and legal for personal use. The website Passeportsante. net has a section describing stretches to do at work and relaxation exercises that can be integrated into your personal relaxation program.

- PasseportSante.net. Baladodiffusion. *Site de PasseportSanté.net*, [online]. http://www. passeportsante.net/fr/audiovideobalado/ Balado.aspx (accessed on May 9, 2013).

There are also a number of paper and digital books on relaxation and general stress management techniques. Here are a few suggestions:

- Bélanger, C., & Beaulieu, J. (2008). *Stress et anxiété, votre guide de survie*. Montreal: Éditions La Semaine.
- Kabat-Zinn, J. (2005). *Wherever You Go, There You Are: Mindfulness Meditation in Everyday Life*. Hyperion.
- Lafleur, J. (2008). *Relaxer : des stratégies pour apprivoiser votre stress*. Montreal: Éditions Logiques.

What should my attitude be with family, friends, and co-workers?

Diabetes can add an element of stress to your interpersonal and professional relationships. Like you, your close friends and family can experience shock, denial, anger, or sadness when learning of your diagnosis, and they may have trouble accepting that the disease is now a permanent part of your life. Some may begin acting like worried parents, trying to tell you what to do and possibly being a bit judgmental in the process (saying things like, "You shouldn't have that dessert," or asking if you've checked your blood sugar). Others might react with denial and make light of the disease ("It's not that serious," "Everyone has to die of something," or "Just take some pills, you'll be fine."). Although they no doubt want to help and to protect you from their own worries about the disease, they may not go about it the right way. If a friend or family member seems to want to control your actions, trivialize your experience, or tempt you to be incautious, you may feel as though they are trying to take control of your disease away from you, and it is normal if you have negative feelings about it.

The important thing is to remain calm and remember that their reactions very likely stem from a lack of information. Try talking to your friends and loved ones about diabetes, being as clear as you can about your needs and expectations. Encourage them to learn about the disease. A helpful book to recommend is:

- Ékoé, J.-M. (2010). *Vivre avec une personne atteinte de diabète*. Montreal: Bayard Canada.

It is important to feel respected, but you might feel that, despite your best efforts, you are not getting the reactions you expected from some people. Do not let it consume you. Speak to them, respect their reactions as much as you can, and turn to the people you feel understand you the best for support.

Some people prefer not to talk about their diabetes in their professional milieu or extended social circle. Nevertheless, it is a good idea to hand-pick a few allies or confidantes who can be ready to help in an emergency. It is your responsibility as someone living with diabetes to create a safe environment for yourself, particularly in the case of an episode of hypoglycemia. Knowing that you have someone you can count on if you need it will help reduce your stress.

What should my attitude be with health professionals?

Your diabetes diagnosis means that your relationship with your doctor and other health professionals is a lifelong partnership. If based on trust and mutual respect, it will be an important factor in your successful control of blood glucose. As in any other important relationship, however, you may at times feel some tension or dissatisfaction with someone on your health care team because of a difference of approach or point of view. Many people with diabetes say that the medical appointments themselves can be very stressful because they are difficult to schedule and usually quite brief, so patients can feel rushed. Getting the most out of them requires that you prepare well beforehand to ensure that your explanations are complete and that your doctor fully understands your situation.

The following book can help deal with these challenges and to understand your doctor not just as a medical professional but as a human being:

- Fortin, B., & Goulet, S. (2012). *Comment améliorer mon médecin? Le patient efficace.* Montreal: Éditions Fidès.

Basically, keeping the lines of communication between yourself and your doctor open, cultivating a trusting relationship, and contributing to your treatment recommendations will lead to a more effective partnership in the treatment of your diabetes. These conditions are essential to maintaining the motivation you need to make the permanent lifestyle changes your doctor recommends.

Bibliography

1 Chaloult, L. (2008). *La thérapie cognitivo-comportementale: Théorie et pratique.* Montreal: Gaëtan Morin.

2 Gregg, J. A., Callaghan, G.M., Hayes, S.C. et al. (2007). Improving diabetes self-management through acceptance, mindfulness, and values: a randomized controlled trial. *Journal of Consulting and Clinical Psychology*, 75, 336–343.

3 Lloyd, C., Smith, J., & Weinger, K. (2005). Stress and diabetes : A review of the links. *Diabetes Spectrum*, 18(2), 121–127.

4 Mercuri, N., Olivera, E. M., Souto, A., Guidi, M. L., & Gagliardino, J. J. (2000). Yoga practice in people with diabetes. *Diabetes Research and Clinical Practice*, 50(Supp. 1), 234-235.

5 Rosenzweig, R., Reibel, D. K., Greeson, J. M., Edman, J. S., Jasser, S. A., McMerty, K. D., & Goldstein, B. J. (2007). Mindfulness-based stress reduction is associated with improved glycemic control in type 2 diabetes mellitus : a pilot study. *Alternative Therapeutic Health Medicine*, 13, 36-38.

6 Sahay, B.K. (2007). Role of Yoga in Diabetes. *Journal of the Association of Physicians of India*, 55, 121-126

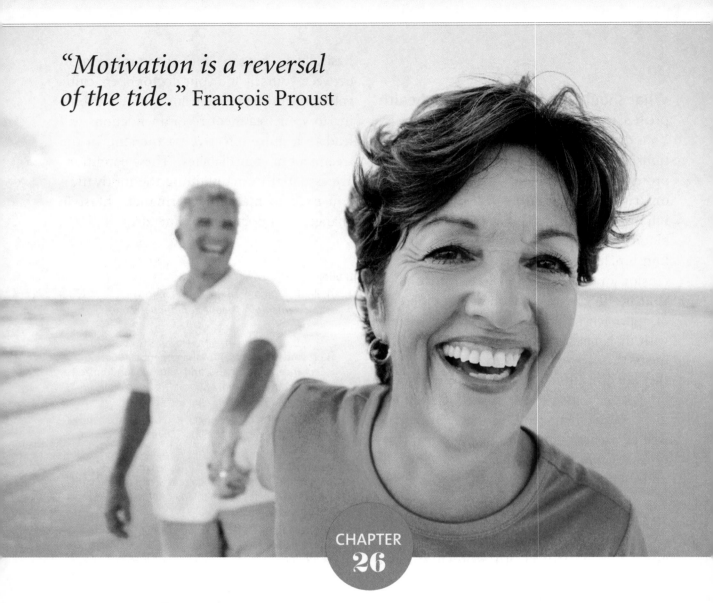

"*Motivation is a reversal of the tide.*" François Proust

The Motivation to Change

As discussed in chapters 24 and 25, the lifelong project of diabetes self-management inevitably involves a number of challenges, including the active acceptance of the disease, the prevention and treatment of diabetes-related mental health issues, and stress management. This chapter discusses the daily actions required to integrate diabetes and its treatment into your life. Although staying up-to-date on any new developments will help ensure that any choices you make are the most likely to promote your health and well-being, knowledge alone is not enough to actually undertake the changes needed. **Motivation** is the key ingredient; it is the motor that gives you the energy you need to start the process of change and the strength to stay the course. This chapter discusses the difficulty of finding the motivation to treat diabetes and introduces a few notions to help reverse the tide of resistance to change and to begin moving in the right direction.

Why is it so hard to get motivated for diabetes self-management?

Finding the motivation, energy and – dare we say – the enthusiasm required to implement a healthy, optimal self-care plan is not easy. This is in large part because diabetes requires self-treatment, a continual monitoring and management of blood glucose levels. People diagnosed with diabetes need to form new habits; day in, day out, they have to make sure that they count their carbohydrates, adjust their nutrition plans, exercise, take medications as needed, refrain from smoking, and manage their stress levels. Even some regular daily chores need adjustment: grocery shopping and cooking meals, for example, require a bit more planning and care than they used to. Restaurant meals have to be considered from a new perspective. And then of course there are the repeated blood glucose readings, regular medical appointments, blood tests every three months, foot care, prescription purchases at the pharmacy, and visits to the ophthalmologist. People who use pen injectors or insulin pumps also have to master the use of their devices, which requires knowledge, focus, maintenance, and time.

The constant effort this requires is indisputable. Everyone with diabetes wishes at some point that they could take a vacation from the disease. It is essentially impossible to take a break from treatment, however. No matter how much you would like to forget it, diabetes will continue to act, quietly, relentlessly, and possibly destructively.

Diabetes is often described as an insidious disease. Whether diagnosed unexpectedly (type 1) or developing slowly (type 2), the failure to treat will lead to complications, but often not until years later. The disease can also be present long before it is diagnosed, causing complications without our knowledge. Whatever the case, it is hard to get motivated for self-treatment when there are no short-term complications or when the complications that do appear could not have been prevented. Diabetes is frequently referred to as an invisible disease, easy to overlook, and therefore requiring extra vigilance. It is easy to see how daily concerns and challenges can take priority and push aside thoughts of diabetes self-care. In addition, the emotions that can arise with respect to diabetes – for example, distress, fear, guilt, anger, or sadness – often cause people to push thoughts about the disease out of their heads and can contribute to the natural resistance to the lifestyle changes that diabetes requires.

Why are people resistant to changing their lifestyle?

"When you change your habits, you change who you are."
Marshall Sylver

Frequently, the lack of willpower and confidence to make concrete changes can be attributed to a belief system that includes certain myths about change itself. A common – and mistaken – belief is that change is always sudden and brutal, when in fact, it is usually a gradual, step-by-step process. Although we may all claim that we are motivated by change, in reality it almost always generates a natural ambivalence between two choices that may at first glance appear to be equal. Ambivalence is not the same as denial or rejection, and it is a perfectly normal reaction.[1] It should be explored to ensure that the choices made are conscious and considered. It can be difficult to let go of the status quo because it represents what is known, safe, stable, and workable. Change forces us to face the unknown, to risk failure, and to lose our bearings.

Your interactions with other people can also strengthen your resistance to change. Unfortunately, despite good intentions, the attitudes of your friends, family members, or medical professionals (whose very role is to promote changes in lifestyle) can create obstacles to healthy transformation. Resistance can result from the tension that is created when someone tries to persuade us that it is critical that we do something that we are clearly not doing. To put it another way, when someone tells us what we could, should, or must do, we tend to balk. When someone warns us that something terrible can happen if we do not change, we may feel a need to rebel because we perceive our autonomy to be at risk.

When you have diabetes, resistance to changing your lifestyle can arise because your objectives are different from those of the health care professionals you deal with. For example, the importance that medical staff places on numbers – blood glucose levels, blood test results – may not be in tune with your priorities as someone living with the disease. Your focus may be on regaining the energy and ability to concentrate that you had before the diagnosis, or on finding a way for your daily activities to what they used to be. Of course, blood glucose control is a way of helping us achieve some of those objectives, but people with diabetes often feel as though their concerns about quality of life are pushed aside or ignored by the medical staff. In such cases, they might provide their blood glucose information or undergo blood tests just "to make the doctor happy" and "avoid being scolded." After a while, they may even feel that there is no point to measuring their blood glucose or doing the tests and simply stop.

How do the myths about diabetes create obstacles to change?

False beliefs about diabetes, often based on incorrect information, rumours, family legends, and cultural perceptions – in short, a lack of knowledge about the disease – can also impede motivation. Prejudices about the disease contribute to poor self-management or even the abandonment of treatment, which is often misunderstood. Sometimes the myths can lead to a course of action that brings about the opposite of the intended effect, and the negative results can in turn compound lack of motivation.

Table 1 presents a list of myths about diabetes that are relatively commonly held by people with the disease and their families and friends. These myths must be challenged. Find information from reliable sources such as a doctor, a specialist in diabetes, diabetes teaching groups, or books on diabetes (like this one). Having a realistic perception of the disease will give you better control over it and motivate you to act in ways that are more likely to lead to success. Table 2 provides a few examples of realistic statements about scientific research on diabetes that can replace the myths listed in Table 1.

Table 1 COMMON MYTHS ABOUT DIABETES

> **Incorrect beliefs based on biased or incomplete information**
>
> 1. If I take my pills to treat diabetes, I can eat whatever I want.
>
> 2. I have a "minor" case of diabetes and my blood sugar is "just a little high," so I don't need treatment.
>
> 3. I can never eat any kind of sugar again.
>
> 4. Most medications to treat diabetes are physically addictive because they are "chemicals" so I should take as little as possible.
>
> 5. Injecting insulin is the same as being a junkie who shoots drugs.
>
> 6. I got diabetes because I ate too much sugar.
>
> 7. Diabetes treated with insulin is much more serious than diabetes treated with oral or injectable antidiabetic drugs.
>
> 8. I no longer have diabetes because my blood glucose is back to normal.
>
> 9. I don't have any symptoms so I don't have the disease.
>
> 10. If I ignore the problems, they will disappear.
>
> 11. Whatever I do, I will develop complications and they will kill me.

What can motivate me to change my habits?

"Ability is what you're capable of doing. Motivation determines what you do. Attitude determines how well you do it."
Lou Holtz

In addition to a realistic understanding of diabetes, two factors contribute to the motivation to change your habits:

1 how important you believe the change to be, and

2 how confident you are that you can successfully change.

To determine your attitude, ask yourself the following:

1 **On a scale of 1 ("not important at all") to 10 ("extremely important"), how important is change to you?**
To explore the ambivalence involved in any type of change, it is useful to understand how important you believe the proposed change to be. When the importance is high, there is a desire for change, and when it is low, there is little conviction that a change will be worthwhile. Of course, the importance you place on a change is often a function of your own priorities and values, including physiological needs (e.g., food), safety needs (e.g., a roof over your head), the

Table 2 REALISTIC BELIEFS ABOUT DIABETES

Beliefs about diabetes based on scientific data

1. If I take pills to treat my diabetes, I can and I should eat a regular, planned amount of carbohydrates.

———

2. Even though I am only in the early stages of the disease, I need treatment to prevent the progression of the disease and complications.

———

3. I need to keep carbohydrates in my diet, but I have to count and manage the amounts. Even though I have diabetes, my body and my brain need a certain amount of carbohydrates to function properly.

———

4. Although medications have some potential known side-effects, they are not addictive. They fill a lack caused by the insufficient production of insulin, which is a vital hormone. All natural physiological activities are "chemical," but that does not mean they are harmful.

———

5. Injecting insulin is evidence of my self-respect because I am giving myself one of the best treatments for diabetes.

———

6. I got diabetes because I have a genetic predisposition to the disease (type 2) or because my immune system turned on my pancreatic beta cells (type 1).

———

7. Diabetes treated with insulin is as serious as diabetes treated with oral or injectable antidiabetic medication. What makes a person's condition more serious is a failure to achieve blood glucose targets, regardless of the treatment.

———

8. Although I am not cured, when I maintain my blood glucose within target levels, my diabetes is well controlled and complications are prevented.

———

9. Even though I don't have any visible symptoms, I still have diabetes.

———

10. If I ignore the problems, complications of the disease will eventually appear.

———

11. If I properly manage my diabetes, I will prevent complications from developing and preserve my quality of life for as long as possible.

———

need to belong (e.g., being a member of a sports team), the need for love (e.g., being part of a couple), the need for self-esteem and accomplishment (e.g., being respected, doing rewarding activities, doing volunteer work). The more self-aware you can be, the easier it will be to understand what is important to you and to re-evaluate your priorities periodically, as you evolve and as challenges present themselves.

2 On a scale of 1 ("not confident") to 10 ("totally confident"), how confident are you that you can change?

The confidence to change can be reinforced by thoughts of your past successes and by recalling the strategies you used to get there. It is also important to look at your more general personal characteristics and resources that can be harnessed in the present situation. Developing self-confidence sometimes means knowing where to start. Your first step should be what you believe you can most easily achieve. Feel free to brainstorm ideas and solutions – this can bring your confidence level up a point or two. It is also a good idea to consider what you would do if faced with an obstacle, so that you will feel more prepared if one arises.

To determine your level of motivation to change for the purpose of managing your diabetes, try answering the following two questions:

- **How important do I consider my health?**
- **How much confidence do I have in my ability to influence my own health?**

In research done on treatment adherence in cases of chronic disease, certain beliefs known as "health beliefs" have been identified as having a positive influence on the adoption of healthy behaviours and on the motivation to change. The more you can develop certain convictions about your health, the more willpower you will have to create healthy habits (e.g., eating well, testing blood glucose regularly, etc.). To evaluate your health beliefs, try answering the following questions:

- Do I consider myself to be vulnerable? Do I really have diabetes?
- Do I believe that diabetes has serious consequences and that complications will develop if I fail to change my lifestyle and habits?

- How much do I believe that my health will benefit if I follow the recommendations of my doctor and other health professionals?
- Do I believe that the benefits of treatment will outweigh the restrictions it imposes?
- Do I feel able to implement the recommendations made by my doctor and other health professionals?

If you answered "yes" to most of these questions, you are motivated to change and have resolved your initial ambivalence. If you answered "no," not only do you lack the conviction that change is important, your confidence in your ability to make the change is low. If that is the case, the following readings can help you work through your ambivalence:

- Fortin, B. (2003). *Se motiver et convaincre.* Montreal: Les éditions CPF.
- Miller, W. R.., & Rollnick, S. (2002). *Motivational Interviewing: Preparing People for Change* (Guilford Press).
- St-Arnaud, Y. (2013). *Comprendre et gérer sa motivation : à quoi carbure l'être humain?* Montreal: Les Éditions Québec-Livres.

How can my family and friends help me get motivated to change my lifestyle?

Essentially, if your family and friends want to help you get motivated, they should not challenge you or refute your arguments; confrontation could in fact produce the opposite result.

The Canadian Diabetes Association recommends the approach known as motivational interviewing to help people with diabetes make changes to their lifestyles.[2] This approach is available to any health professional. Its goal is to elicit "change talk" from the person with diabetes – in other words, to encourage you to develop and articulate the advantages of changing in your own words (Miller & Rollnick, 2006). As a person with diabetes, it is to your advantage to become aware of the motivational power of speaking positively about change. Put simply, talking positively to yourself about the changes you wish to make can be very encouraging.

Open-ended questions (e.g., "What kind of change would you like to make?", "What would the advantages of changing be for you?") are used to elicit a description of the drawbacks of not changing and the benefits of changing, as perceived by the person with diabetes. Motivational interviewing does not attempt to convince you to change or to impress upon you that change is urgent; rather, it respects your pace and seeks to understand the importance

that you place on change, while emphasizing your strengths and capacities. The process involves discussion that is empathetic and that does not test, analyze, congratulate, disapprove, or alarm. Advice is given only if asked for explicitly. Questions about the advantages and disadvantages of the current situation and the desired situation can help you project yourself into the future. Your feelings of personal effectiveness are supported and encouraged as you describe how you see yourself achieving your goals, the solutions you envisage, and the steps you wish to take.

What are the stages of change?

"No matter how far you go, no matter how high, you must begin your journey with a simple step." Shitao

Understanding how change happens is a crucial step your journey, even when your motivation is low or you have relapsed into old habits. Knowing what change is helps us recognize the stage we have reached (*see Table 3*). The road between point A and point B is not straight but full of twists and turns, and you might sometimes feel as though you are moving in circles. The following illustration presents a spiral model of the steps toward change.[5] The image illustrates how change does not happen in one step but takes place only after practice, trial and error, and a repeated feeling of being back at square one. It shows how even relapses constitute steps toward change, with each one bringing us a step closer to our objective as we learn from our mistakes and refine our plan, becoming more aware potential obstacles and unforeseen events. Nothing is black or white: as you persevere and accept each step on your path towards growth, achievement and failure coexist. The ideal attitude to prevent diabetes burnout has been defined by Polonsky:[4]

1 Clearly identify the barriers to diabetes self-management so that you can overcome them more easily.
2 Stay motivated, and forgive yourself for not being perfect; do not exhaust yourself with impossible goals.[3]

Understanding the five stages of change as a spiral can help you identify actions that can propel you from one stage to the next. Table 3 presents ideas for actions you can perform to help yourself take the next step.

"Success is falling down seven times and getting up eight." Japanese proverb

A **relapse** is a return to one of the five prior stages of change, where the process begins again until the next relapse, and so on until termination. After each relapse, which requires cycling through the process again, we find ourselves at a higher stage in the ascending spiral. The learning that takes place each time equips us with more wisdom and experience as the journey towards termination continues. Much like trip-

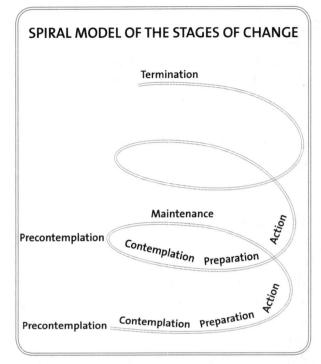

From Prochaska, J. O., Diclemente, C. C., & Norcross, J. C. (1992). "In search of how people change: applications to addictive behavior" *American Psychologist* 47(9), page 1104.

ping can teach us to walk better, a relapse is an opportunity to learn how to steady ourselves as we move towards our goals.

Table 3 DESCRIPTION OF THE STAGES OF CHANGE

Stages	Description	Actions
Precontemplation	• No! I have no intention of changing my behaviour.	• I remain open to change. • I look for more information that can make me more aware of the importance of changes that might be good for me.
Contemplation	• Yes, I am starting to consider making some changes over the next six months, but…	• I identify the obstacles to change. • I evaluate the drawbacks and benefits of the change. • I ask for help from the people around me
Preparation	• I need some tips! I've made the decision to make a change over the next month.	• I make a plan and establish clear objectives. • I make a verbal commitment to my doctor or a loved one.
Action	• I take action. • I am experimenting and have been implementing a change for less than six months.	• I look for support when I am feeling the most vulnerable such as during vacation or stressful periods. I do my best to plan for the unexpected, and I revise my plan as I go.
Maintenance	• I'm used to it. I've made a change and I have been maintaining it for at least six months.	• I give myself healthy rewards when I obtain my objectives (e.g., a massage, an evening out).
Relapse	• I am stuck in one of the loops of the spiral of change. I am going back to one of the previous five stages. I feel like I am going backwards.	• I go back to the habits I had before the change. I forget. I cheat.
Termination	• I am so used to it that I now do it without thinking and I no longer relapse.	• I have permanently and harmoniously integrated the change into my life.

Prochaska, J. O., Diclemente, C. C., & Norcross, J. C. (1992) In Search of How People Change: Applications to Addictive Behavior. American Psycholo gist 47(9), 1102–1114.

How can I ensure that my objectives have the best possible chances of success?

"Goals are not only absolutely necessary to motivate us. They are essential to really keep us alive." Robert H. Schuller

During the preparation stage of change, before you are ready to take action, you must set your objectives. Since the 1960s, business managers have been breaking down their general objectives into smaller, more specific objectives. Short-term actions are thus harmonized and integrated, as the long-term goal comes more and more into focus. Following this model, to increase the probability of termination and success, it is best to reflect and define your objectives according to the **SMARTS** model. In other words, your objectives must be:

- **Specific:** The objective must be clear. For example, instead of saying vaguely, "I will eat more regularly," be more precise: "I will eat three meals a day, five days a week. In other words, from Monday to Friday, I will have breakfast at 8:00 a.m., lunch at noon, and dinner at 5:00 p.m. On weekends, I will have regular meals at 9:00 a.m., 1:00 p.m., and 6:00 p.m."
- **Measurable:** It is easier to evaluate our progress if we have concrete goals to measure, such as "I aim to eat 50 grams of carbohydrates in the morning, in liquid form if needed, even if I have no appetite." It is hard to determine whether an vague goal (e.g., "I will eat more in the morning") has been met.
- **Attainable:** You must sincerely agree with the objective you set. When you begin the process of change, choose the objective that is the most motivating or that you want the most. Do not begin with an objective set by others or by events. Some authors have described this criterion as being an "Achievable" goal.
- **Realistic** Take small steps that are in keeping with the circumstances. Small successes accumulate to create a solid foundation as you move toward your ultimate success. Reassess your objective if there are any changes in circumstances.
- **Time-bound:** Draw up a schedule. Determine when you will begin, plan a period of experimentation, and consider how often you will have to reassess your progress and your plan to meet your objective. You may have to redefine your objective even more precisely.
- **Supported:** Assess the support – whether social or emotional – that you will need to achieve your goal. It can be from your family, friends, colleagues, or your medical team. It can also be what is referred to as "instrumental" support in the form of a book, an information brochure, a carbohydrate counting device, or even a watch alarm. Be creative.

What are some objectives that can motivate me to adopt new habits to treat my diabetes?

"The future depends on what we do in the present." Mahatma Gandhi

In Western society, it is generally agreed that exercising more and eating better are the most difficult changes for people with diabetes to make. Taking antidiabetic drugs or insulin is apparently less problematic because it involves less of a profound change in everyday habits. This section provides a few concrete strategies and objectives to encourage the adoption of new habits.

To exercise more:

- **Make physical activity part of another activity.** Walk your dog or take your bike to work, for example.
- **Begin slowly.** It's better to walk ten minutes a day than not walk at all.
- **Remember the benefits of exercise.** Physical activity is an excellent way to lower stress, fight depression, and protect against heart disease. It also helps people with diabetes control blood glucose.
- **Write it in your agenda.** Plan exercise the way you plan work or social activities.
- **Be flexible.** Do exercise that is the most accessible, the most time effective, the most convenient for your budget, and the best adapted to your abilities.

- **Enjoy it.** Try different kinds of physical activity to discover what you enjoy the most.
- **Share your physical activities with other people.** Find partners to go on walks, play tennis, or go bird-watching with.

To eat well:

- **Draw up a clear and realistic nutrition plan with a dietitian.**
- **Change your environment to make it easier.** For example, do not buy cookies if you know you will not be able to resist.
- **Put things in perspective when results are not what you hoped.** For example, use your glycated hemoglobin results in addition to your weekly blood glucose readings to assess the impact of weight loss on your control over your diabetes.
- **Do not be too strict.** Moderation is key. Depriving yourself of food can lead to the urge to abandon your new habits altogether and eat even more.
- **Focus on the new lifestyle habits you hope to acquire instead of the ones you want to quit.**
- **Seriously consider reorganizing your life.** If your everyday life seems boring and eating is your only pleasure, vary your sources of personal enjoyment and satisfaction. For example, begin volunteering or find a new hobby.
- **Be assertive.** This is especially important if you are someone who finds it hard to say no. Think of yourself before you think of others, and be sure you are meeting your own needs.

Motivation is one of the essential elements in the healthy self-management of diabetes. As you make your way through the process of change, there will be ups and downs – this is unavoidable, even desirable. Take pride in your actions that are motivated by your values and convictions. Making these types of changes in your life is one of the best ways to evolve, reach your full potential, and create a life that meets your needs while preserving your quality of life, your mental health, and your physical health. The risk is well worth it.

1 Beckman, H. (2012). *The Diabetes Motivation Book: Change One Thing at a Time with the Science of Willpower*. Middleton, WI: Daniel Meinen.

2 Robinson, David J. et al. (2013). Canadian Diabetes Association Clinical Practice Guidelines Expert Committee. Canadian Diabetes Association 2013 Clinical Practice Guidelines for the Prevention and Management of Diabetes in Canada: Chapter 18: diabetes and mental health. Can J Diabetes 2013;37(suppl 1):S87-S92. Accessed at http://www.guidelines.diabetes.ca.

3 Joslin Diabetes Center. *Avoid Diabetes Burnout*. Consulted at: http://www.joslin.org/managing_your_diabetes_596.asp (accessed May 13, 2013).

4 Polonsky, W. H. (1999). *Diabetes Burnout: What to Do When You Can't Take It Anymore*. Alexandria, VA : American Diabetes Association.

5 Prochaska, J. O., Diclemente, C. C., & Norcross, J. C. (1992). In search of how people change: applications to addictive behaviors. *American Psychologist*, 47(9), 1102-1114.

6 Welch, G., Rose, G., & Ernst, D. (2006). Motivational interviewing and diabetes: What is it, how is it used, and does it work? *Diabetes Spectrum*, 19(1), 5-11.

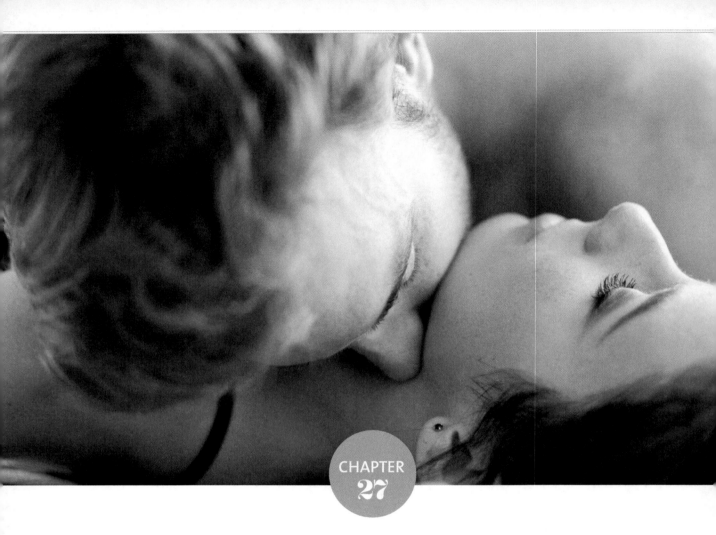

Sex and Family Planning

Can diabetes affect the sex lives of people with diabetes?

Diabetes can cause problems affecting sexuality in both men and women. In women, the problems are less obvious and generally don't directly impede sexual intercourse; as a result, they have been studied less and are less understood. In men, chronic high blood glucose can make it difficult to achieve and maintain erection and thus hamper the ability to have satisfactory sexual intercourse. This is known as erectile dysfunction.

MEN

Do all men with diabetes suffer from erectile dysfunction?

No. Erectile dysfunction is not an inevitable side effect of diabetes. On average, it affects between 35% and 45% of men with the disease. If you experience erectile dysfunction at any given time, talk to your doctor. In addition to having a negative effect on your quality of life, in some cases the condition is also a sign of cardiovascular disease. Your doctor will help you get control of the situation.

How does diabetes cause erectile dysfunction?

Over the long term, hyperglycemia can cause two problems:

- nerve damage, also known as neuropathy;
- a thickening and hardening of the arteries, which can hamper circulation (atherosclerosis).

These two conditions, either separately or combined, can result in the partial or complete inability to achieve erection (erectile dysfunction).

Poorly controlled diabetes generally affecting a man's health can also cause erectile dysfunction. In such cases, correcting hyperglycemia usually enables a return of normal sexual function.

When men with diabetes have erectile dysfunction, is it always caused by the disease?

No. Erectile dysfunction can be multifactorial (have a number of causes) and can frequently be attributed to something other than diabetes. Erectile dysfunction in men with diabetes may have nothing to do with their disease. For example, it can be due to:

- lifestyle: tobacco, alcohol, drugs;
- heart disease, high blood pressure, high cholesterol;
- consequences of surgery or radiation therapy to the prostate, urinary tract, colon, or rectum;
- certain medications;
- certain hormonal issues resulting in lowered testosterone;
- specific psychological issues.

Can men with diabetes prevent erectile dysfunction?

Yes. The risk of erectile dysfunction can be reduced by:

- keeping blood glucose levels as close to normal as possible;
- following a meal plan;
- quitting smoking, if applicable;
- stopping or decreasing alcohol consumption, if applicable;
- controlling high blood pressure and any blood lipid abnormalities;
- taking prescribed medications.

How is erectile dysfunction assessed?

The following tests are performed to assess erectile dysfunction:

- Doppler test to measure penile blood flow;
- electromyography (EMG) of the penis to measure neurological conductivity;
- blood tests to measure the levels of certain hormone (e.g., testosterone);
- evaluation of nocturnal erections; the occurrence of nocturnal erections suggests that the issue may have a psychological origin;
- if the above tests are negative or if the couple requests, evaluation by a psychologist or sex therapist.

Is there treatment for erectile dysfunction in men with diabetes?

Yes. Your doctor can help you find an effective treatment. The first step to finding the appropriate treatment is to identify the problem.

1 Better control of blood glucose is usually helpful.

2 Any potential hormonal problems should be corrected.

3 Any medications potentially affecting sexual function should be eliminated, if possible.

4 In many cases, drugs can be used to induce erection and make full sexual intercourse possible.

The medications currently available are:

- oral medications such as Viagra®, Cialis® or Levitra®;
- Muse®, a prostaglandin suppository inserted into the urethra;
- Caverject®, a prostaglandin injection at the base of the penis;

5 In cases of severe organic erectile dysfunction, a penile prosthetic device can be used.

6 Finally, sex therapy might be useful, either to help the person adapt to the challenges or to resolve any psychological issues at the root of the problem.

WOMEN

Are there any risks associated with pregnancy in women with diabetes?

Yes. To limit the risks, women with diabetes are strongly encouraged to plan their pregnancy with their health care team. For the most part, the risks are related to poor control of blood glucose before and during pregnancy.

When diabetes is actively treated and pregnancy is adequately planned, the risks of complications related to diabetes are greatly reduced.

In most cases, diabetes is properly controlled, there are no complications, and women give birth to healthy babies. Remember that your health care team is there to guide you through all the changes brought on by your pregnancy. They can help you control your diabetes properly while preventing it from taking up too much space in your life. In this way, you can ensure that your pregnancy is safe for both you and your child and that you are able to fully appreciate this joyful time.

The risks that arise during pregnancy, which are primarily related to less-than-optimal blood glucose control, can be categorized into two types: risks to the mother and risks to the baby.

Increased risks to the mother:

- spontaneous miscarriage;
- more frequent hypoglycemia with a possible decrease in the associated symptoms;
- more pronounced hyperglycemia with a risk of acidosis in women with type 1 diabetes;
- rapid aggravation of complications of diabetes that were present before the pregnancy (e.g., risk of progression in previously untreated kidney damage or retinopathy);
- high blood pressure and preeclampsia (pregnancy complication characterized by increased blood pressure, protein in the urine, and œdema of the legs, hands and face), which may require inducing labour, even before term;
- cæsarean section or more difficult vaginal birth (because of the weight of the baby).

Risks to the baby:

- Deformities, particularly of the fetal heart and kidneys: deformities occur primarily if the mother's diabetes is poorly controlled at the time of conception and in the first months of the pregnancy;
- Premature birth;
- Greater-than-average weight at birth (macrosomia): baby weighing more than 4 kg (9 lbs) at birth;
- Difficulty breathing at birth;
- Hypoglycemia at birth: usually because of the woman's poorly controlled diabetes late in the pregnancy;
- Jaundice during the first few days of life;
- Fetal or perinatal death: because the treatment of women with diabetes has been improving, newborn mortality has considerably decreased. Its incidence is still higher for women who have poor control of their diabetes, however.

What should women with diabetes do to prevent complications associated with pregnancy?

Generally, complications can be avoided by the strict control of blood glucose levels, careful planning of the pregnancy, and close follow-up by a multidisciplinary team in a specialized health care centre.

To maximize the chances of a smooth pregnancy, women with diabetes are strongly urged to consult their doctors before they stop using birth control with the intention of getting pregnant.

Before getting pregnant, it is very important to:

1 evaluate and treat any complications that could worsen during pregnancy, particularly issues affecting the eyes;

2 control blood glucose before pregnancy to limit the risk of congenital deformities:

- women are advised to achieve and maintain an A1C less than or equal to 7.0% before conception, ideally maintaining it around 6.0%;

- to reach this goal, you might need to modify or increase your medication. Your health care team can help you. Even if you cannot reach this goal, remember that any decrease in A1C increases your chances of having a healthy baby. Women whose A1C is above 10%, however, should continue to use contraception and postpone their pregnancy until they have reached their targets;

3 with the help of your doctor, ensure that your medication is safe for the fetus during the pregnancy;

- Some medications (e.g., angiotensin-converting enzyme for high blood pressure and statins to lower blood cholesterol) are not recommended during pregnancy. Your doctor should stop your prescription or substitute them before conception or very early in the pregnancy;

4 quit smoking, if applicable, and practice healthy habits including balanced nutrition and regular exercise (3 to 4 sessions a week for a total of 150 minutes);

5 maintain a healthy weight (a BMI between 18.5 and 25 kg/m^2 is ideal). Women who are overweight (BMI ≥ 25) are recommended to reach a healthy weight before getting pregnant or to lose at least 10% of their body weight. Even if the ideal weight is not reached, a 10% weight reduction has a positive effect on fertility and reduces the risk of complications during pregnancy;

6 begin taking vitamin supplements, including 5 mg of folic acid daily, ideally three to six months before the pregnancy.

Only after meeting these targets can a woman with diabetes realistically expect to have a safe pregnancy.

What should blood glucose targets be before and during pregnancy?

Before pregnancy, to reach the target A1C of less than or equal to 7.0%, ensure that your blood glucose before meals is under 7.0 mmol/L most of the time. To help you better control your blood glucose, your doctor may suggest increasing or modifying your treatment. Some women with type 2 diabetes could be advised to begin insulin therapy before getting pregnant to ensure better blood glucose control. It should be remembered, however, that stricter control of blood glucose through oral medications or insulin can increase the risk of hypoglycemia. Essentially, women with diabetes who plan to get pregnant and who need to take hypoglycemic drugs are advised to monitor their blood glucose more closely to avoid hyperglycemia and hypoglycemia.

During pregnancy, target blood glucose levels are lower (*see table on page 271*). They may appear quite strict, but they are necessary because:

- normally, a pregnant woman's blood glucose drops during pregnancy and for physiological reasons remains lower until delivery; and
- hyperglycemia considerably increases the risk of deformities, obstetric complications, and macrosomia (large for gestational age). A big baby can make delivery more difficult or even risky.

Therefore, fasting blood glucose between 6.0 and 6.5 mmol/L, while perfectly appropriate when a woman is not pregnant, is too high during pregnancy.

In addition, hormone levels increase throughout pregnancy, affecting blood glucose and requiring constant adjustments to treatment. Women should therefore set lower target blood glucose levels as soon as they learn they are pregnant, since this will optimize the health and development of the fetus. They also need to learn how to deal with more difficult-to-manage blood glucose levels.

Blood glucose should be monitored more closely during pregnancy. Women who are used to checking once or twice a day should increase the number of readings to one or two hours after every meal. Pregnant women with diabetes can use this time as an opportunity to develop healthier life habits, with nutrition playing a central role. A dietitian or nutritionist should be consulted both before the pregnancy and early on in the first trimester to revise the meal plan. In addition to adapting to changes in carbohydrate needs, the new meal plan can also integrate revisions to protein, iron, folic acid and calcium intakes.

In summary, controlling blood glucose levels during pregnancy is often very different from controlling them before pregnancy. Pregnant women should expect a period of transition, during which they must learn how their bodies are reacting to certain nutrients, activities, and

BLOOD GLUCOSE TARGETS FOR WOMEN WITH DIABETES		
	Before and after pregnancy	During pregnancy
Fasting and pre-meal blood glucose	4.0 to 7.0 mmol/L	3.8 to 5.2 mmol/L
Blood glucose 1 hour after a meal	No target	5.5 to 7.7 mmol/L
Blood glucose 2 hours after a meal	5.0 to 10.0 mmol/L	5.0 to 6.6 mmol/L
Glycated hemoglobin (A1C)	≤ 7.0%*	No target

* ≤ : Less than or equal to

stress levels. Moreover, pregnancy hormones influence blood glucose control, potentially making it more complicated. Do not hesitate to contact your health care team to adjust your treatment quickly.

Is breastfeeding possible for women with diabetes?

Of course. Diabetes has no impact on breastfeeding. In addition to the demonstrated benefits for babies, breastfeeding can help mothers keep blood glucose under control and lose the weight they gained during pregnancy. Many women develop hypoglycemia during or following a feeding, however, especially at night. It is therefore important that you monitor your blood glucose more frequently while breastfeeding and have a snack before or during the feeding. Your nutritionist can help you draw up a meal plan to help you avoid hypoglycemia, while also ensuring that your breastfeeding is successful and that you can gradually shed the weight you gained during pregnancy.

Finally, just like pregnant women, women who are breastfeeding should check whether the drugs they are taking are safe. Insulin is completely safe for the baby because it is not absorbed into the breast milk. Some drugs, however, including some oral antidiabetics, are absorbed into the breast milk in small quantities. See your doctor to revise and adapt your medication for as long as you are breastfeeding.

Does the treatment of diabetes change quickly after a woman gives birth?

Yes. Almost immediately after giving birth, the need for insulin decreases considerably. The concentration of pregnancy hormones decreases very rapidly and insulin sensitivity improves. Regardless of the type of diabetes you have, your treatment will change the day after you give birth.

Gradual return to initial medication

Type 1 diabetes

Women with type 1 diabetes will not need much insulin in the first few days after giving birth. As the days go by, insulin doses should be increased gradually to reach the levels taken before pregnancy. Since the body's insulin needs change quickly in the first weeks after giving birth, new mothers should stay in touch with their health care team during this period.

Type 2 diabetes

Women with type 2 diabetes who took insulin before they got pregnant will very likely continue the same treatment but at lower doses than what they were taking while pregnant. If they were on oral antidiabetic therapy before they got pregnant, the treatment might be changed to insulin for as long as they are breastfeeding and afterwards return gradually to oral antidiabetics.

What are the risks of a child developing diabetes if one of the parents has the disease?

If one of the parents has type 1 diabetes, the long-term risk of the child developing diabetes is 5%. The risk is a little higher if the father is the parent with the disease.

If one of the parents has type 2 diabetes, the long-term risk of the child developing diabetes is 25%.

Are there any methods of contraception that should be avoided or favoured by women with diabetes?

There are no contraceptive methods specifically designed for women with diabetes. However, like all women, a woman with diabetes should carefully choose her contraceptive method with her health in mind, since some may present a higher risk of complications.

The choice should be guided by her age, how long she has had diabetes, how well she controls it, the known complications, whether she smokes, the number of prior pregnancies, the effectiveness of the contraception, and above all the preferences of the woman and her partner.

Effective contraceptive methods

1 Hormonal contraceptives:
 • Combined oral contraceptive pills contain two hormones, estrogen and progestin. They are very effective, but for some women they can have an impact on blood glucose control and carry certain risks for the blood vessels. There is also a skin patch (Evra®) and a vaginal ring (Nuva Ring®) that release a combination of estrogen and progestin;
 • Low-dose progestin pills contain a small amount of progestin (e.g., Micronor®). They are effective if taken every day at the same time and have little impact on blood glucose;
 • Intramuscular injections of progestin (Depo-Provera®) every three months is a very effective method with no impact on blood glucose or the blood vessels. However, weight gain and a loss of bone density have been reported by some groups of women using this method.
2 Intra-uterine devices (IUDs) are very effective and carry no additional risk of infection if the woman with diabetes has good control over her blood sugar. In addition to being effective, IUDs with progestin (Mirena®) are safe because they have no effect on blood sugar or the blood vessels.
3 Barrier methods such as condoms, diaphragms and spermicides can be used safely by women with diabetes.

Can women with diabetes use emergency oral contraception (the "morning-after pill")?

Yes. Emergency oral contraception used after unprotected sexual intercourse is not contra-indicated for women with diabetes. It is not recommended as a regular contraceptive method, however. Emergency oral contraceptives are taken in one of the following ways:
 • a 100 µg dose of ethinylestradiol (an estrogen) combined with 500 µg of levonorgestrel (a progestin) as soon as possible after intercourse, with a second dose 12 hours later (for example, two doses of two Ovral® tablets); or
 • one dose of 750 µg of levonorgestrel (Plan B®) as soon as possible after intercourse and a second dose 12 hours later.

Emergency oral contraception must be prescribed by a doctor. In Quebec, they may also be prescribed by pharmacists.

Are sterilization methods available to women with diabetes and their partners?

Sterilization is an option for people with diabetes, just as it is for anyone does not want to have children and wishes to use a permanent method of contraception.

The options are:

- tubal ligation, for women;
- vasectomy, for men.

Can menopausal women with diabetes take hormones?

Yes. Menopausal women with diabetes can take hormones in the form of estrogen, either with or without progestin.

However, it has recently been shown that combined hormone therapy (estrogen and progestin) is associated with a minimal but significant risk of breast cancer, thrombophlebitis (blood clots), strokes, and heart disease, especially if the treatment is taken over several years.

Therefore, menopausal women should take hormones (estrogen and progestin) only if the symptoms are difficult to manage on a daily basis (e.g., hot flashes) and only for a maximum of four years, on average. The hormones should be taken in the lowest dose that still effectively controls the symptoms. Once

the symptoms are gone, the woman can be weaned off the hormones and eventually stop hormone therapy altogether.

When deciding whether to take estrogen, the following high-risk situations should be taken into account, if relevant:

- a history of thrombophlebitis;
- a history of cerebrovascular problems, specially in women who smoke;
- a history of breast cancer.

If an estrogen-based treatment is contraindicated, in most cases other options are available. Talk about it with your doctor.

In short, hormone therapy is safe for menopausal women as long as they take into account any potential risks related to estrogen and can receive follow-up. The choice to take hormone therapy should be based on whether the symptoms of menopause are present and whether the therapy would improve quality of life.

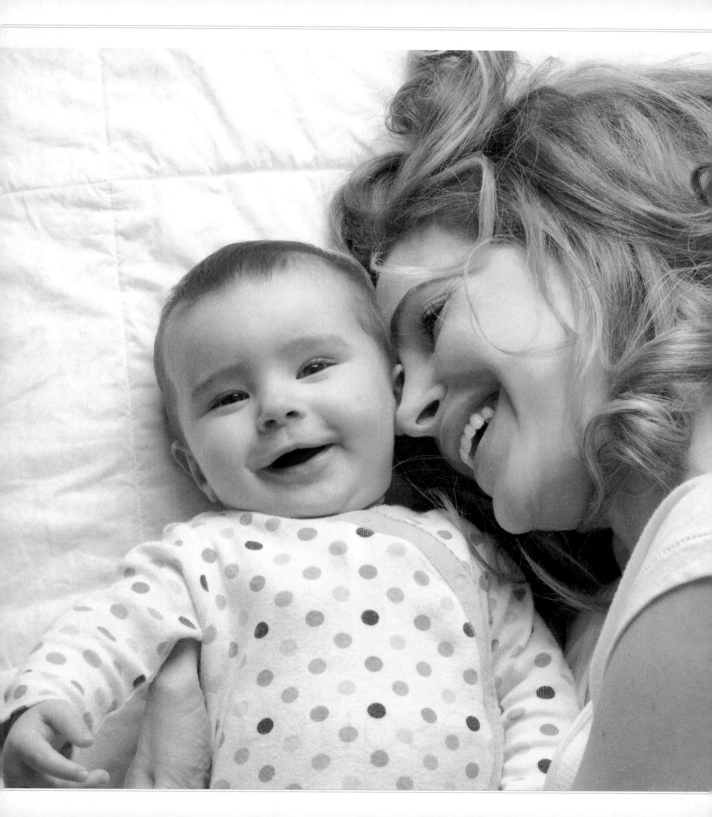

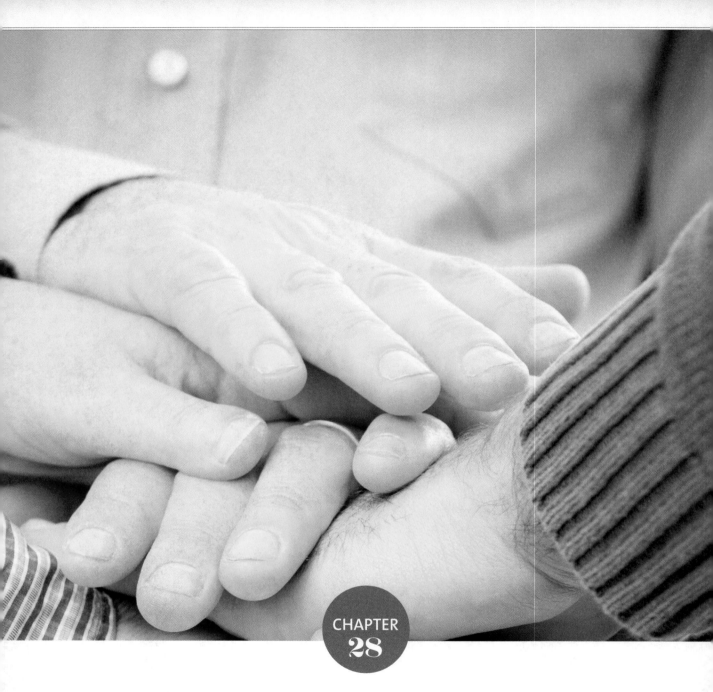

CHAPTER
28

Resources

This book was written by the multidisciplinary team of the Diabetes Day Unit of the CHUM Hôtel-Dieu Hospital.

The CHUM Hôtel-Dieu diabetes day unit opened its doors in March 1995 in response to a need for diabetes education, research, and development.

Every week, the Diabetes metabolic day unit welcomes dozens of people with diabetes for individual meetings with a multidisciplinary team of endocrinologists, nurses, dietitians, and psychologists.

Our team also offers group training sessions giving people an opportunity to learn more about every aspect of diabetes, helping people with diabetes become more independent with respect to their illness.

The following training programs are offered to people with diabetes:
- one-day intensive course
- one-day refresher course every six months (after the initial training)

Everything is offered free of charge, and every person with diabetes who take part receives a copy of the book *Understand Your Diabetes and Live a Healthy Life*.

Anyone who is interested can contact:

Diabetes Day Unit
CHUM Hôtel-Dieu
3840 Saint-Urbain St.
Montreal QC H2W1T8
Tel.: 514 890-8141

There are a number of other diabetes teaching centres accessible through the health network. See the Diabetes Québec magazine *Plein Soleil* or the Diabetes Québec website for a list of these centres.

PHYSICAL ACTIVITY

What exercise services and facilities are available to people with diabetes?

**Amicale des diabétiques des hôpitaux
Notre-Dame et Maisonneuve-Rosemont**
(aquafitness, gentle conditioning,
group walking)
2065 Alexandre-de-Sève St.
9th floor, ste. Z-9903-4
Montreal QC H2L 2W5
Tel.: 514 890-8000, ext. 25358
Email: amicale.diabetique.chum@ssss.gouv.qc.ca
Website: www.amicaledesdiabetiques.com

Centre ÉPIC
**(preventive medicine and physical activity
centre of the Montreal Heart Institute)**
5055 Saint-Zotique St. E
Montreal QC H1T 1N6
Tel.: 514 374-1480
Fax: 514 374-2445
email: info@centreepic.org
Website: www.centreepic.org

Clinique de kinésiologie
CEPSUM—Université de Montréal
2100 Édouard-Montpetit Blvd.
Montreal QC H3C 3J7
Tel.: 514 343-6256
Fax: 514 343-2467
Websites:
www.kinesio.umontreal.ca
www.cepsum.umontreal.ca

**Centre de santé et de services sociaux
Jeanne-Mance**
(CSSS Jeanne-Mance)
Health motivation education centre
2260 Parthenais St.
Montreal QC H2K 3T5
Tel.: 514 521-2361, ext. 2319
Website: www.csssjeannemance.ca

**Fédération québécoise de la marche and
Marche-Randonnée magazine**
4545 Pierre-de-Coubertin Ave.
Montreal QC H1V 0B2
Tel.: 514 252-3157 or toll-free 1 866 252-2065
Fax : 514 252-5137
Website: www.fqmarche.qc.ca
(see "Nos organismes affiliés" page for a list of
walking clubs)
Email: infomarche@fqmarche.qc.ca

Outdoor recreational activity groups — for the more active types
- www.actionpassion.com
- www.ecoaventuremonde.com
- www.azimutaventure.com/
- www.bougex.com
- www.horizonroc.com/
- www.aventuriers.qc.ca
- www.cycloconcept.ca
- www.cyclonature.org
- www.detournature.com
- www.karavaniers.com
- www.groupeoxygene.qc.ca
- www.passionaventure.com

Kino-Quebec
- www.kino-quebec.qc.ca
- www.actimetre.qc.ca (adult physical activity assessment software and recommendations)

SOCIOECONOMIC SUPPORT

What kind of socioeconomic support is available?

WELFARE ACCESS
People with diabetes who are eligible for welfare receive an additional $20 per month. Speak with the agent responsible for your file for further information.

Solidarité sociale,
Bureau des renseignements et plaintes
Tel.: toll-free 1 888 643-4721

FAMILY ALLOWANCE
An extra $167 per month is added to the family allowance for parents with a dependent child who has diabetes. The request for the supplement must be filled out and signed by the pediatrician.

Régie des rentes du Québec
Tel.: 514 864-3873 or 1 800 667-9625
(benefits for handicapped children)

TAX CREDIT
People with chronic diseases requiring daily care may be entitled to a federal tax credit.

LOANS AND BURSARIES
- Full-time CEGEP or university students with diabetes are reimbursed for the cost of their medication.
- Students must make a loan and bursary request at their school's financial aid office and follow the steps for the program.

INSURANCE

What factors should people with diabetes consider when taking out insurance?

IMPORTANT FACTS

- Insurance taken out before the diagnosis of diabetes remains in force under the same terms.
- When a new insurance application is made, people with diabetes must undergo a medical assessment to determine their new level of risk. There is no overarching policy for people with diabetes; each individual case is considered on its own merits.
- In the case of mortgage life insurance, the benefit is usually not available if the diabetes is pre-existing or if the disease is diagnosed before the renewal of the policy.

GROUP INSURANCE

- People with diabetes receive compulsory coverage, like all other employees. People with diabetes may take out optional coverage with no additional premium if the request is made before the imposed deadline. Beyond the deadline, coverage is usually refused.
- In many cases, when a person leaves a job, the group insurance policy can be converted into an individual insurance policy.

INDIVIDUAL LIFE INSURANCE

- People with diabetes should shop around and talk to several insurance companies before signing a contract. Every insurer has its own method of evaluation.
- There are many possible types of insurance for people with diabetes:
  - Additional premiums, which can vary widely. In some cases they increase from one year to the next. Premiums depend on the individual's risk assessment
  - Health option flat rates, where the admissibility and maintenance of the coverage depends on criteria determining how well the diabetes is controlled.

ASSOCIATIONS

What associations provide support for people with diabetes?

Canadian Diabetes Association
1400-522 University Ave.
Toronto, ON M5G 2R5
Tel.: 1 800 226-8464
Email: info@diabetes.ca
Website: www.diabetes.ca
Magazine: *Diabetes Dialogue*
Website: www.diabetes.ca/dialogue

American Diabetes Association
1701 North Beauregard St.
Alexandria VA 22311
USA
Tel.: 1 800 342-2383
Website: www.diabetes.org
Magazine: *Diabetes Forecast*
Website: www.forecast.diabetes.org

Diabetes Québec
8550 Pie-IX Blvd., ste. 300
Montreal QC H1Z 4G2
Tel.: 514 259-3422 or 1 800 361-3504
Email: info@diabete.qc.ca
Website: www.diabete.qc.ca
Magazine: *Plein soleil*

BLIND OR AMBLYOPIC

What services are offered to people with diabetes who are blind or amblyopic?

Philips Lifeline
Remote surveillance (two-way vocal communicator)
774 Décarie Blvd., ste. 100
Saint-Laurent, Quebec H4L 3L5
Tel.: 514 735-2101 or 1 877 423-9700
Website: www.lifeline.ca

MAB-Mackay Rehabilitation Centre
7000 Sherbrooke St. W.
Montreal QC H4B 1R3
Tel.: 514 488-5552
Fax: 514-489-3477
Website: www.mabmackay.ca

Institut de réadaptation en déficience physique du Québec
525 Wilfrid-Hamel Blvd., Wing J
Quebec QC G1M 2S8
Tel.: 418 529-9141
Fax: 418 529-3699
Website: www.irdpq.qc.ca

Canadian National Institute for the Blind
120 Crescent St., ste. 201-1
Montreal QC H3A 2A9
Tel: 514 934-4622 or 1 800 465-4622
Fax: 514 934-2131
Email: quebec@cnib.ca
Website: www.cnib.ca

Institut Nazareth et Louis-Braille
1111 Saint-Charles St. W
Longueuil QC J4K 5G4
Tel.: 450 463-1710 or 1 800 361-7063
Fax: 450 463-0243
Website: www.inlb.qc.ca

CD for the visually impaired
Diabetes Québec
Plein soleil magazine
Tel.: 514 259-3422 or 1 800 361-3504

Blood glucose metres
Oracle from Tremblay Harrison, with speech synthesizer
Tel.: 1 866 829-7926
Website: www.oraclediabetes.com

Regroupement des aveugles et amblyopes du Montréal métropolitain
5215 Berri St., ste. 200
Montreal QC H2J 2S4
Tel.: 514 277-4401
Fax: 514 277-8961
Email: infor@raamm.org
Website: www.raamm.org

Service québécois du livre adapté
475 de Maisonneuve Blvd. E.
Montreal QC H2L 5C4
514 873-4454 or 1 866 410-0844
Website:
www.banq.qc.ca/portal/dt/sqla/sqla.htm

DIABETES QUÉBEC

What services are offered by Diabetes Québec?

Diabetes Québec
8550 Pie-IX Blvd., ste. 300
Montreal (Quebec) H1Z 4G2
Tel.: 514 259-3422 or toll-free 1 800 361-3504
Email: info@diabete.qc.ca
Website: www.diabete.qc.ca

Diabetes Québec is a non-profit association bringing people with diabetes and health professionals together. Its mission is to educate, sensitize, and prevent, and its work focuses on four aspects: educating, funding research, defending the rights of people with diabetes, and providing services. Some of the services it provides are free, while others are offered at a nominal price:

- *Plein soleil*, a magazine featuring useful information about diabetes, provides a list of its forty affiliated organizations;
- lectures;
- educational materials (books, brochures, and the DVD "*Foot Care for Diabetics*");
- training tailored to specific groups of people with diabetes and health professionals;
- InfoDiabetes, an information service:
  514 259-3422, ext. 233
  or toll-free 1 800 361-3504
  or by email at infodiabete@diabete.qc.ca.

BEREAVEMENT

What bereavement services are available to people with diabetes?

Vie nouvelle
(information about the grieving process and discussion groups)
Verdun Hospital
4000 LaSalle Blvd., Suite 5114
Montreal QC H4G 2A3
Tel.: 514 362-1000, ext. 2883
Fax: 514 362-7402

CHILDREN

What services are offered to children with diabetes?

Camp pour enfants diabétiques de l'est du Québec
4500 Henri-Bourassa Blvd., ste. 20
Quebec QC G1H 3A5
Tel.: 418 523-6159
Email: info@cedeq.org
Website: www.cedeq.org

Juvenile Diabetes Research Foundation
615 René-Lévesque Blvd., ste. 330
Montreal QC H3B 1P5
Tel.: 514 744-5537 or 1 877 634-2238
Fax: 514 744-0516
Email: montreal@jdrf.ca
Website: www.jdrf.ca

The Diabetic Children's Foundation and Camp Carowanis
306 St. Zotique St. E.
Montreal, QC H2S 1L6
Tel.: 514 731-9683 or 1 800 731-9683
Fax: 514 731-2683
Email: carowanis@diabete-enfants.ca
Website: www.diabetes-children.ca

MEDICAL IDENTIFICATION TAGS

Where can I get a medical identification bracelet or pendant?

Jewellery stores

Canadian Medic-Alert Foundation
2005, Sheppard Ave. E,
ste. 800
Toronto ON
M2J 5B4
Tel.: 416 696-0267 or 1 800 668-6381
Website: www.medicalert.ca

Pharmacies

FEET

What foot care services are available?

Association des infirmières et infirmiers en soins de pieds du Québec
3850 Jean-Talon St. W., ste. 99
Montreal QC H3R 2G8
Tel.: 514 344-7212 or toll-free 1 800 771-9664
Fax: 514 344-0766
Email: info@aiispq.qc.ca
Website: www.aiispq.org

Podiatric assessment and treatment clinic for patients with diabetes (diabetic foot)
CHUM Hôtel-Dieu
3840 Saint-Urbain St.
Montreal QC H2W 1T8
Tel.: 514 890-8151 (make an appointment)

Ordre des podiatres du Québec
300 Jean-Talon St. E., Anjou
Montreal QC H1M 3N8
Tel.: 514 288-0019 or 1 888 514-7433
Website: www.ordredespodiatres.qc.ca

DRIVER'S LICENCES

What factors should people with diabetes consider when getting a driver's licence?

IMPORTANT FACTS
- Diabetes can cause problems that affect visual sharpness and field of vision. Obviously, vision plays a fundamental role in driving an automobile.
- Driving is a privilege, not a right to be taken for granted or bestowed without reservation.
- The SAAQ (Société de l'assurance automobile du Québec) establishes the rules governing the acquisition and holding of this privilege. These rules are based on a person's ability to drive in a manner that is safe for himself and for all others. The state of the driver's health is taken into account.

MEDICAL ASSESSMENT
- A medical assessment form is sent out to people with diabetes at varying intervals.
- The report must be filled out by the person's doctor and/or optometrist within the time frame specified (three months).
- The SAAQ bases its decision on this medical opinion. It places more weight on functional limitations than on the diagnosis itself.

The SAAQ medical assessment takes into account how well the diabetes is controlled.

HYPOGLYCEMIA AND DRIVING

- Hypoglycemia can compromise the ability of a person with diabetes to drive safely. It occurs most often in people with diabetes who are treated with insulin and, less frequently, in people taking medications to stimulate the production of insulin (sulfonylureas,meglitinides).

NECESSARY PREVENTIVE MEASURES INCLUDE:

- Always check your blood glucose before driving and follow the recommendations in the chapter on hypoglycemia.
- Always have rapidly absorbed sugars nearby.
- Avoid driving for long periods without a break.
- Never skip meals or snacks.
- Carry an emergency food supply in case a meal is delayed.

LEGAL OBLIGATIONS

The law provides the following:

- Holders of a driver's licence are under a legal obligation to inform the SAAQ of any disease or change that is related to their physical and mental health when they first apply for their permit and within 30 days of any change in their health. Knowingly providing false or misleading information is an offence and can lead to driver's licence suspension and a fine.
- Holders of a driver's licence are under a legal obligation to respond to a request for a medical report within the specified time.

Any person providing false or misleading information is guilty of an offence and may be subject to prosecution. A false declaration renders the driver fully responsible, which could have serious repercussions in the event of an accident.

SAAQ (SOCIÉTÉ DE L'ASSURANCE AUTOMOBILE DU QUÉBEC)

For more information:
Service de l'évaluation médicale
P.O. 19500
Quebec QC G1K 8J5
Tel.: 418 643-5506 or
toll-free 1 800 561-2858
Website: www.saaq.qc.ca

PROFESSIONALS

DIETITIAN SERVICES

What nutritional resources are available to people with diabetes?

DIETITIANS

Ordre professionnel des diététistes du Québec
2155 Guy St., ste. 1220
Montreal
QC H3H 2R9
Tel.: 514 393-3733 or toll-free 1 888 393-8528
Website: www.opdq.org

BOOKS ABOUT DIABETES AND NUTRITION

- Isabelle Galibois, *Le diabète de type 1 et ses défis alimentaires quotidiens* (Quebec: Les Presses de l'Université Laval, 2005).

COOKBOOKS WITH CARBOHYDRATE COUNTS

- Anne Lindsay, *Smart Cooking: Quick and Tasty Recipes for Healthy Living* (Canadian Cancer Society, 1997).
- Bonne Stern, *Heart Smart* (Random House Canada, 2006).
- Anne Lindsay, in collaboration with Denise Beatty of the Canadian Medical Association, *Anne Lindsay's New Light Cooking* (Random House Canada, 2006).
- Manon Poissant, Céline Raymond & Josée Rouette, *La nouvelle cuisine santé* (Éditions Stanké, 1998).*

- Karen Graham, *Diabetes Meals for Good Health* (Robert Rose, in collaboration with the Canadian Diabetes Association, 2012).
- Manon Robitaille & Daniel Lavoie, *Le dessert se fait léger* (Éditions Diabète Québec, 2007).
- Nicole Delisle, Mélanie Forget & Sylvie Larouche, *Diabétiques, les sucres et pourquoi pas !* (Profil Santé Diététique inc. et Association Diabète du Québec, 2001).
- Nicole Delisle, Mélanie Forget & Sylvie Larouche, *Les sucres... Question d'équilibre* (Éditions Profil Santé Diététique Inc., 2007).
- Helen Bishop, et al., *Eat Well, Live Well: The Canadian Dietetic Association's Guide to Healthy Eating*, (Macmillan of Canada, 1990).*
- Katherine E. Younker, *The Best Diabetes Cookbook* (published in cooperation with the Canadian Diabetes Association, Robert Rose, 2005).
- Geneviève O'Gleman, *Rapido-presto 150 recettes santé en 30 minutes* (Éditions Semaine (La), 2009).
- *Qu'est-ce qu'on mange?* Vol. 4. (Cercle des fermières du Québec, 1997).
- Various authors, *Simplement délicieux* (Éditions du Trécarré, 2007).
- *Cooking Light Magazine, Cooking Light: Fresh Food Fast* (Time Home Entertainment, 2009).

*The books marked with an asterisk are out of print and not available in bookstores, but can be found in libraries or in used bookstores.

WEBSITES ON DIABETES AND NUTRITION
Recipe analyzer
- Dieticians of Canada:
  http://www.eatracker.ca/recipe_analyzer.
  aspx?lang=en
- Carbohydrate calculator (advanced method)
  www.diabete.qc.ca (use the search bar)
- "L'Épicerie": television show on Radio-
  Canada
  www.radio-canada.ca/emissions/l_
  epicerie/2012-2013
- Extenso, Centre de référence sur la nutrition
  humaine (information on human nutrition)
  www.extenso.org
- Fédération des producteurs maraîchers du
  Québec (federation of market gardeners of
  Quebec)
  www.legumesduquebec.com
- Canada's Food Guide
  www.hc-sc.gc.ca/fn-an/food-guide-aliment/
  index-eng.php
- Passeport santé
  www.passeportsante.net
- SOS cuisine
  www.soscuisine.com

Nutritional value of foods
- CalorieKing
  www.calorieking.com
- Canadian Nutrient File
  http://webprod3.hc-sc.gc.ca/cnf-fce/
- Nutrient values of some common foods
  http://www.hc-sc.gc.ca/fn-an/alt_formats/
  pdf/nutrition/fiche-nutri-data/
  nvscf-vnqau-eng.pdf

WEBSITES FEATURING RECIPES WITH CARBOHYDRATE COUNTS
- Canadian Diabetes Association
  http://www.diabetes.ca/diabetes-and-you/
  recipes/
- American Diabetes Association
  http://tracker.diabetes.org/recipe/
- Diabetes Québec
  http://www.diabete.qc.ca/html/
  alimentation/recette.html (only in French)

MOBILE APPLICATIONS (APPS)
- Guide resto par Diabète Québec
- GluRefPro: Based on data from Health
  Canada, GluRefPro gives you the carbohydrate
  count for over 5000 food items and their carb
  factors, no matter where you are.

Available on iTunes App Store and Google Play
for Android.

NURSING SERVICES

What nursing care resources are available to people with diabetes?

NURSES

Ordre des infirmières et infirmiers du Québec
4200 Dorchester Blvd. W.
Westmount QC H3Z 1V4
Tel.: 514 935-2501 or toll-free 1 800 363-6048
Fax: 514 935-1799
Email: inf@oiiq.org
Website: www.oiiq.org

Info-Santé
CLSC (Quebec community health centres) telephone help line, available 24 hours a day to provide answers to health questions. Dial 811.

CLSCs (community health clinics). All are open from 8 a.m. to 4 p.m.

MEDICAL SERVICES

How can I get medical assistance?

Collège des médecins du Québec
2170 René-Lévesque Blvd. W.
Montreal QC
H3H 2T8
Tel.: 514 933-4441 or toll-free 1 888 633-3246
Fax: 514 933-3112
Website: www.cmq.org

DOCTORS

My family doctor:

_____

☎ _____

My endocrinologist:

_____

☎ _____

On-call endocrinologist
at my hospital:

_____

☎ _____

PHARMACY SERVICES

How can I get help from a pharmacist?

Ordre des pharmaciens du Québec
266 Notre-Dame St. W, ste. 301
Montreal QC
H2Y 1T6
Tel.: 514 284-9588 or toll-free 1 800 363-0324
Website: www.opq.org

Any pharmacy

Régime public d'assurance-médicaments (Quebec) (public drug insurance program)
- Contact the Régime de l'assurance maladie du Québec
  Tel.: 1 888 435-79999
  Website: www.ramq.gouv.qc.ca

PHARMACISTS

My pharmacist:

☎ _____

My pharmacy

☎ _____

MENTAL HEALTH SERVICES

What psychological/mental health services are available to people with diabetes?

PSYCHOLOGISTS OR PSYCHOTHERAPISTS
Ordre des psychologues du Québec – Public and private resources
1100 Beaumont Ave., ste. 510
Mont-Royal QC
H3P 3H5
Tel.: 514 738-1881 or toll-free 1 800 363-2644
Website: http://www.ordrepsy.qc.ca/en/index.sn
http://www.ordrepsy.qc.ca/en/public/trouver-un-professionnel/index.sn

Referral through CSSS and CLSC - Adults
A request for psychological services can be made with the Centre de Santé et de Services Sociaux (CSSS, Health and Social Service Centre) in your area with a doctor's referral or from your Centre Local de Services Communautaires (CLSC, Local Community Service Centres). Ask for access to adult mental health or psychosocial services. For the contact information of the CSSSs or CLSCs in Montreal, refer to the following websites (consulted on May 10, 2013).
http://www.santemontreal.qc.ca/en/chercher-une-adresse/#csss
http://www.santemontreal.qc.ca/en/chercher-une-adresse/#clsc

Specialized clinics/centres (for depression, anxiety, eating disorders, alcohol, drug or gambling additions) - Montreal area

- **Anxiety and mood disorders**
  Institut universitaire en santé mentale de Montréal
  Hôpital Louis-Hippolyte LaFontaine
  7401 Hochelaga St.
  Montreal QC
  H1N 3M5
  Tel.: 514 251-4000, ext. 3029
  Website: http://www.iusmm.ca/hopital/usagers-famille/acces-aux-services.html
  Services are accessed through the evaluation and brief consultation program (programme Évaluation et interventions brèves, or PEIB) (via emergency or with a doctor's reference).

- **Mood disorders**
  Douglas Mental Health University Institute
  6603-6605 LaSalle Blvd.
  Montreal QC
  H4H 1R3
  Tel.: 514 888-4469
  Fax: 514 888-4460
  Websites: http://www.douglas.qc.ca/page/mood-disorders-program
  http://www.douglas.qc.ca/page/evaluation-liaison-module
  Schedule: Monday to Friday, 8:30 a.m. to 4:30 p.m.

To access services, a reference from a health professional is required (including a complete physical examination).

- **Eating Disorders Program**
  Douglas Mental Health University Institute
  6603-6605 LaSalle Blvd.]montreal QC
  H4H 1R3
  Tel.: 514 761-6131, ext. 2895
  Fax: 514 888-4085
  Website: http://www.douglas.qc.ca/section/troubles-de-l-alimentation-146?locale=en
  Schedule: Monday to Friday, 8:30 a.m. to 4;30 p.m.
  To access services, a medical reference from a health professional is required (you will have to undergo a complete physical exam).

- **Centre Dollard-Cormier**
  950 de Louvain St. E
  Montreal QC
  H2M 2E8
  Tel.: 514 385-1232
  Website: ww.centredollarcormier.qc.ca
  Schedule: Monday to Friday, 8:00 a.m. to 8:00 p.m.
  For Urgence-Toxicomanie, a helpline for drug-related emergencies, call 514 288-1515, 24 hours a day, 7 days a week.

Support groups (depression, anxiety, eating disorders) – Montreal area

- **Anorexia and Bulemia Quebec (ANEB)**
  5500 Transcanadienne
  Pointe-Claire QC
  H9R 1B6
  Tel.: 514 630-0907 or 1 800 630-0907
  Email: info@anebquebec.com
  Website: http://www.anebquebec.com/
  html/en/home/home.html

- **Groupe d'entraide G.E.M.E. (stress, panic attacks, anxiety, burnout, depression) – Head office**
  1085 Ste-Foy Blvd., ste. 232
  Longueil QC
  J4K 1W7
  Tel.: 450 332-4463 or 1 866 443-4363
  Email: info@geme.qc.ca
  Website: http://www.geme.qc.ca/news.
  php#.UfWFL41wq6U
  Schedule: Monday to Friday, 9:30 a.m.
  to 12:00 p.m. and 1:00 p.m. to 5:00 p.m.

- **La clé des champs (support network for people with anxiety disorders**
  2226 Henri-Bourassa Blvd., ste. 100
  Montreal QC H2B 1T3
  Tel.: 514 334-1587
  Fax: 514 461-1351
  Email: lacle@lacledeschamps.org
  Website: http://lacledeschamps.org/english/
  anxiety-disorders-montreal/

- **Phobies-Zero**
  P.O. Box 83
  Sainte-Julie QC
  J3E 1X5
  Tel.: 450 922-5964
  Fax: 450 922-5935 (telephone first)
  Website: http://www.phobies-zero.qc.ca/
  Schedule: Monday to Friday, 9: a.m.
  to 4:00 p.m.
  The telephone helpline is available from
  Monday to Friday, 9:00 a.m. to 9:00 pm.,
  at 514 276-3105 or 1 866 922-0002

- **Revivre (depression, anxiety, bipolar disorder)**
  5140 St-Hubert St.
  Montreal QC
  H2J 2Y3
  Tel.: 514-REVIVRE(738-4873) or
  1 866-REVIVRE
  Fax: 514 529-3081
  Email: revivre@revivre.org
  Website: http://www.revivre.org/home.php
  Schedule: Monday to Friday, 9:00 a.m.
  to 5:00 p.m.

- **Tel-Aide (telephone support line for people in distress, available 24 hours a day)**
  514 935-1101

SEX THERAPISTS

What resources are available for assistance with sexual issues related to diabetes?

Association des sexologues du Québec
7400 Crémazie Blvd. E., ste. 709
Montreal QC
H2P 2X2
Tel.: 514 270-9289
Fax: 514 270-6251
Website: www.associationdessexologues.com

Sexual Dysfunction Unit at the CHUM
Hôpital St-Luc
Édouard-Asselin Building, 5th floor
264 René-Lévesque Blvd. E
Montreal
QC H2X 1P1
Tel.: 514 890-8351

Brochure from Diabetes Quebec:
Édith Fanny Morin, *Diabète et sexualité féminine : Que se cache-t-il derrière le rideau ?*

WEBSITES

What are some useful websites about diabetes?

- Canadian Food Inspection Agency (information on food labelling and advertising) www.cfia-acia.agr.ca
- Public Health Agency of Canada http://www.phac-aspc.gc.ca/cd-mc/diabetes-diabete/index-eng.php
- American Diabetes Association www.diabetes.org
- American Dietetic Association www.eatright.org
- Canadian Diabetes Association www.diabetes.ca
- Société francophone du diabète www.sfdiabete.org
- CDC Diabetes Public Health Resource www.cdc.gov/diabetes
- Diabetes Québec www.diabete.qc.ca
- Diabetes Insight www.diabetic.org.uk
- Diabetes Health Library http://diabeteshealthlibrary.com
- European Association for the Study of Diabetes www.easd.org
- International Diabetes Federation www.idf.org
- Forum for Injection Technique (FIT) www.fit4diabetes.com

- Joslin Diabetes Center
  www.joslin.harvard.edu
- Juvenile Diabetes Research Foundation Canada
  www.jdfc.ca
- Diabetes in Canada
  http://www.hc-sc.gc.ca/hc-ps/dc-ma/diabete-eng.php
- Dietitians of Canada
  www.dietitians.ca
- Medline plus: diabetes
  www.nlm.nih.gov/medlineplus/diabetes.html
- National Diabetes Education Program
  www.ndep.nih.gov
- National Institute of Diabetes & Digestive & Kidney Diseases
  www2.niddk.nih.gov/

SMOKING

What services are offered to people with diabetes who want to quit smoking?

Centre d'abandon du tabagisme

Free assistance and personalized support is available everywhere in Quebec.

- Speak to a specialist on the telephone on the J'Arrete telephone support line:
  1-866-jarrete or 1 866 527-7383.
- Resources to help you keep your resolve are available online at www.jarrette.qc.ca.
- Meet with a professional at a Centre d'abandon du tabagisme (centre for quitting

smoking) nearest you for personalized services to help you quit.

- At the CHUM: For an appointment, call 514 890-8226 or for information 514 890-8000, ext. 15983

WORK

What workplace concerns should people with diabetes keep in mind?

People with diabetes should tell people at their workplace about their disease.

- The *Quebec Charter of human rights and freedoms* protects people with diabetes against any and all discrimination.
- People with diabetes should be as candid as possible with their employer and a few select colleagues, keeping in mind workplace context (for example, it is a good idea to inform people of what to do in the event of serious hypoglycemia).

Some jobs or professions should be avoided.

- People with diabetes are not advised to take certain jobs such as airplane pilot or high-voltage line workers, etc.
- Some jobs can be difficult for people with diabetes. Some examples include garbage collector (increased risk of infection), cook (difficult to follow the meal plan), and jeweller (requires excellent eyesight).

Workplace behaviour

- At first, employers or colleagues may change the way they interact with a co-worker who has diabetes. This is to be expected and should be a temporary stage of the adaptation process.
- Like everyone else, people with diabetes have the fundamental right to be full members of society. Work is one of the most important tools to help achieve personal growth and self-realization.
- The International Association of Machinists - Center for Administering Rehabilitation and Employment Services (**AIM CARES**) can help you. This association offers a free specialized job search service.
  750 Marcel-Laurin Blvd., ste. 450
  Saint-Laurent, Quebec H4M 2M4
  Tel.: 514 744-2944 or 514 744-2613
  Email: emploi@aimcroitqc.org
  Website: www.aimcroitqc.org

Play up your strengths

People with diabetes who are looking for a job should make the most of the skills and strengths they have had to develop because of their disease. These qualities – self-discipline, consistency, perseverance, dedication to a healthy lifestyle, to name but a few – are without a doubt advantages for someone competing on the job market.

TRAVEL

What services are offered to people with diabetes who want to travel?

Travel Health Clinics in Canada
Public Health Agency of Canada
Website: http://www.phac-aspc.gc.ca/index-eng.php

Clinique Santé-Voyage Saint-Luc (Saint-Luc travel health clinic)
1001 Saint-Denis St., 6th floor
Montreal QC
H2X 3H9
Tel.: 514 890-8332
Fax: 514 412-7309
Email: info@santevoyagesaint-luc.com
Website: www.santevoyage.com

Diabetes Québec
Travel Guide for People with Diabetes
Paper version: order by telephone at
514 259-3422 or 1 800 361-3504
Mobile app: available on iTunes App Store and Google Play for Android

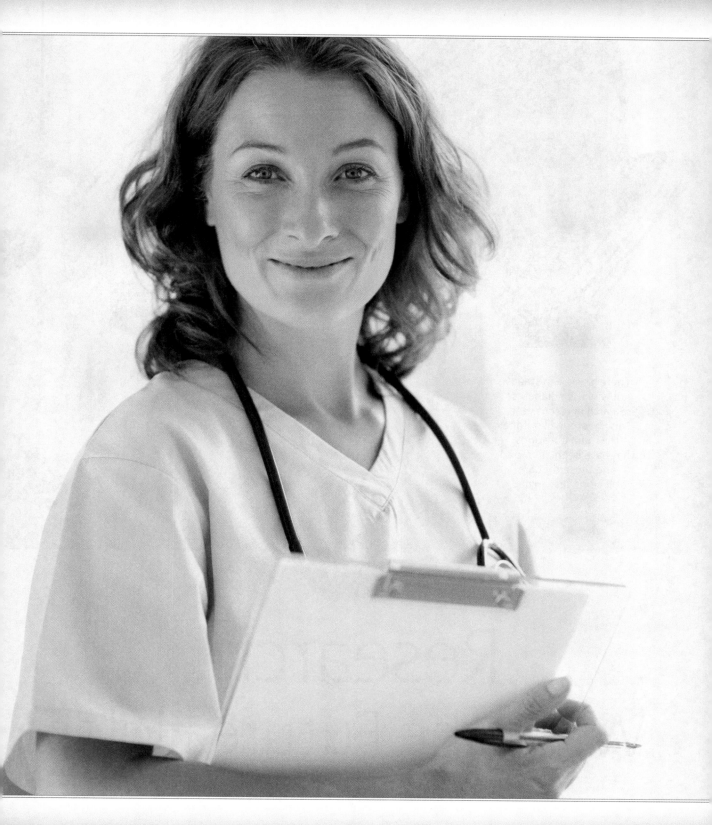

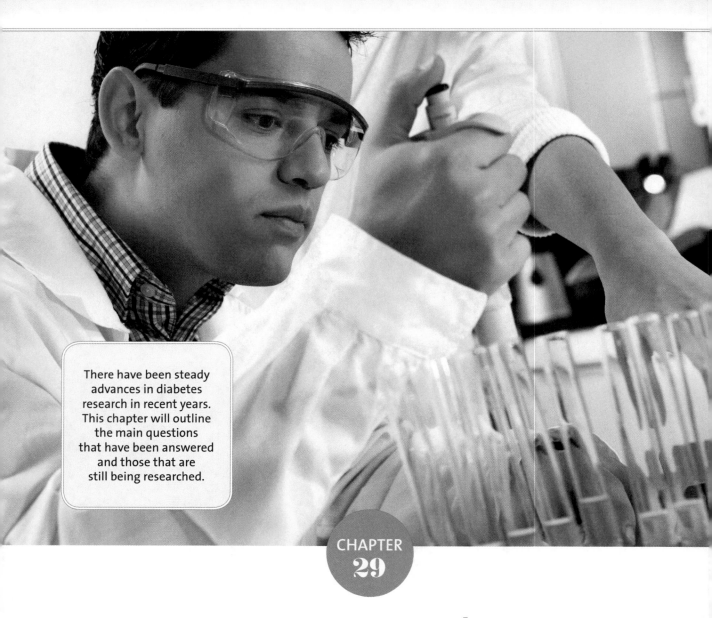

There have been steady advances in diabetes research in recent years. This chapter will outline the main questions that have been answered and those that are still being researched.

Research:
What the Future Holds

What causes type 1 or "juvenile" diabetes?

Alterations in the pancreatic beta cells, caused by environmental factors such as a viral infection, can lead to the body's loss of recognition of its own cells. Mistaking them for foreign cells, the body produces antibodies to destroy them. The capacity to create antibodies against one's own cells has a genetic component, and these antibodies can be detected approximately five years before the disease develops.

Can diabetes be prevented?

A number of different methods have been attempted to prevent people at high risk from developing the disease.

- attempts to use treatments blocking the production of antibodies as soon as they appear and treatments using insulin injections or orally administered doses have so far failed to prevent type 1 diabetes, but this avenue still holds some promise;
- an international nutritional study currently underway is trying to determine whether early introduction of solid foods or cow's milk to young children at risk could influence the risk of developing type 1 diabetes later on;
- there is currently research underway into the genes involved in the development and progression of diabetes, whether type 1 or type 2. Teams from Montreal have made a

number of discoveries in this area. Gene KIAA0350, which codes for a protein that binds molecules containing sugar, has been associated with type 1 diabetes. Several genes (including TCF7L2) that are involved in the development and functioning of pancreatic beta cells and in metabolic mechanisms have variants that create a predisposition to type 2 diabetes in approximately 70% of cases.

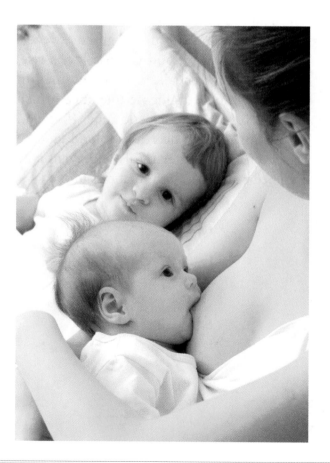

What is the cause of type 2 diabetes?

There are two major factors involved in the development of type 2 diabetes: insulin resistance (meaning that a great deal more insulin is required to maintain normal blood glucose levels) and a decrease in the capacity of pancreatic cells to produce insulin. In most cases, insulin resistance precedes the development of diabetes by several years. As long as the pancreatic cells can compensate by producing more insulin, blood glucose levels remain normal. It is only once the pancreatic cells are no longer able to compensate and insulin production decreases that blood glucose levels increase. At first, blood glucose levels rise, especially after meals, in a phenomenon known as impaired glucose tolerance, which characterizes the prediabetic state. If insulin production further decreases, blood glucose rises even higher after meals and eventually even before meals. This is diabetes proper.

What factors contribute to insulin resistance?

Susceptibility to insulin resistance and a lowered capacity for insulin production are in part hereditary. Excess weight and a lack of physical activity contribute to insulin resistance and an increased risk of developing diabetes. Research has shown that efforts to reduce insulin resistance in people who are glucose intolerant (in particular, regular exercise and weight loss) can significantly reduce the risk of developing diabetes.

What approaches can help prevent type 2 diabetes?

The ideal is to intervene as early as possible. This can be quite a challenge, however, because in some cases, the increased risk of developing diabetes begins even before birth if the fetus is exposed to unfavourable conditions in utero. Gestational diabetes in the mother and low birth weight are possible risk factors for the development of diabetes as an adult. Various approaches have been shown to be effective in the prevention of type 2 diabetes:

- improved nutrition and greater physical activity (lifestyle modifications);
- various pharmacological agents, including metformin, have been associated with some benefits. No drugs have been approved for diabetes prevention in Canada, however;

- bariatric surgery, or weight-loss surgery, which involves reducing the size of the stomach or inducing malabsorption.

What factors are responsible for the complications of diabetes?

In the 1990s, two major studies definitively confirmed that the microvascular complications of diabetes (retinopathy, nephropathy, neuropathy) are related primarily to high blood glucose levels over many years. The first study, an American-Canadian trial published in 1993 (DCCT), followed 1440 patients with type 1 diabetes. The second, a British trial published in 1998 (UKPDS), followed 4209 patients with type 2 diabetes. Both found that diabetes, whether type 1 or type 2, should be aggressively treated and that the complications of diabetes can be prevented by keeping target blood glucose levels as close to normal as possible.

A number of more recent studies have confirmed the importance of optimal blood glucose control to avoid complications, particularly microvascular complications (retinopathy, nephropathy, neuropathy). These more recent studies have not demonstrated any short-term benefits of intensive blood glucose treatment on cardiovascular health, however; it may be that these benefits will appear only in the long term, after more than ten years of follow-up.

The STENO-2 study demonstrated that intensive treatment of multiple factors including blood glucose, blood pressure, and cholesterol not only reduces microvascular complications (retinopathy, nephropathy, neuropathy), but also lowers mortality rates and decreases the number of cardiovascular events (infarcts, stroke). The study also confirmed the importance of controlling all the risk factors (cholesterol, blood pressure, diabetes, etc.). Long-term follow-up in the DCCT and STENO-2 studies has shown that the benefits continue for several years after the end of intensive treatment.

Can complications be prevented?

The prevention of the complications of diabetes represents one of the great research challenges. Thanks to our improved understanding of the physiopathological mechanisms responsible for complications, a few studies are currently evaluating the effectiveness of specific drugs in the prevention of complications regardless of blood glucose control.

The major role of high blood glucose levels in the development of the complications of diabetes has already been described here. A number of studies have shown that high blood sugar is associated with an overproduction of an enzyme known as protein kinase C, and that this enzyme is involved in the development of complications. Pharmaceutical companies have developed a kinase C protein inhibitor and demonstrated that it can prevent complications in animals with diabetes. Studies on humans have not shown any noticeable benefits.

Researchers are also beginning to study drugs inhibiting growth factors that play a role in the development of retinopathy (pegaptanib, ranibizumab and bevacizumab). Fibrates, which are used to reduce triglyceride levels, have also demonstrated a slight reduction of the risk of the progression of retinopathy.

Human studies are currently underway to assess whether drugs acting on incretins (DPP-4 inhibitors, GLP-1 analogues) are likely to reduce cardiovascular complications. Results will be available as of 2014. Vigour trial has already reported not cardiovascular benefit but also no harm.

Large-scale studies of the cardiovascular safety of all of the new antidiabetic treatments are currently needed. They are now underway and are mandated by the various regulatory authorities (e.g., HPB, FDA).

Is diabetes easy to control?

The DCCT and UKPDS studies have shown that normal blood glucose levels are difficult to achieve. In Canada, the DICE study looked at patients followed by front-line doctors and showed that close to 50% of people with type 2 diabetes do not attain their recommended treatment targets. These studies and others (including ADVANCE and BARI-2D) have also demonstrated that treatment often needs to be intensified with supplemental drugs and, if necessary, insulin.

While the use of already existing medications can certainly help control the disease, we must continue to look for new treatments to make these crucial goals easier to achieve.

How can the gradual deterioration of blood glucose control be prevented?

Methods to preserve pancreatic beta cell function and residual insulin secretion are also important topics of research at the moment. In animals, thiazolidinedione and incretin drugs have been shown to have a positive effect on beta cells by decreasing cell death and increasing cell proliferation.

Are there any new treatments for diabetes?

A number of antidiabetic drugs and new techniques are currently being studied or will soon be available in Canada. The following are worth noting:

- drugs that slow gastric emptying, giving time to the pancreas to react, such as pramlintide (Symlin®);
- long-acting GLP-1 analogs that can be administered once or twice a week. Some GLP-1 analogues (incretin-based treatments) are already marketed in Canada, but they require daily injections;
- inhibitors of glucose transport in the kidney that increase the elimination of glucose through the urine: for example, canagliflozine was approved in the United States in late March 2013;
- new oral agents stimulating insulin secretion (GP40R);

- new insulins with specific action profiles: very long-acting insulins (e.g., degludec) may reduce the risk of hypoglycemia and offer more flexibility with regard the time of injection; ultra-rapid acting insulins are also available;
- new technical procedures to connect an insulin pump to a continuous blood glucose monitor, creating a kind of artificial pancreas.

Although the progress in pancreas transplants have been slow, there have been spectacular technological advances in recent years in the development of an artificial pancreas.

What challenges do transplants present?

- **Pancreas transplants** have been successfully executed in various Canadian hospitals, including the CHUM Notre-Dame Hospital. The two major obstacles to pancreas transplants are the shortage of donors and the side effects of anti-rejection drugs.
- More recently, progress has been made in the **transplantation of the islets of Langerhans**, a procedure involving the injection of insulin-making pancreatic cells. An innovative group of researchers from Edmonton, Alberta have improved the technique of isolating the islets of Langerhans and used new combinations of anti-rejection drugs (without cortisone). These transplants are performed under

local anesthesia on an out-patient basis. A catheter is inserted into the portal vein entering the liver and a syringe is used for the injection. The isolation technique enables the recovery of only 20% of the islets, however, and two and sometimes even three donor pancreases are required to obtain a sufficient amount of islets of Langerhans for the transplant. The destruction of the islets over time also means that the cure offered by this technique is temporary. The problem of donor shortage is therefore all the more acute. Improved techniques for isolating the islets, however, should provide a partial solution to this problem.

- New avenues are also being explored in the search for transplantable cells that produce and secrete insulin. Thanks to **genetic engineering techniques**, cells from the intestine or liver can now be genetically programmed to produce insulin. Interesting results have been obtained in animals, but a lot of work remains before this technique can be used on humans.

- In recent years, there has been a great deal of discussion about embryonic stem cells and stem cells from adult human bone marrow. Stem cells have the innate capacity to develop into any type of mature cell, including insulin-producing pancreatic cells. Experiments in this area have only just begun, but they have been very encouraging.

What are the benefits of diabetes research?

It is clear that diabetes is a huge challenge due to the rapidly increasing prevalence of the disease, caused primarily by the aging of the population and the ever-rising number of people with weight problems. Research has led to new pharmacological and technological advances, however, promising not only that it will be easier to control blood glucose in the future, but also that the disease and its complications might one day actually be cured. Diabetes research, which involves participation of a number of Canadian researchers, is being carried out all over the world and continues to bring a great deal of hope to people with diabetes

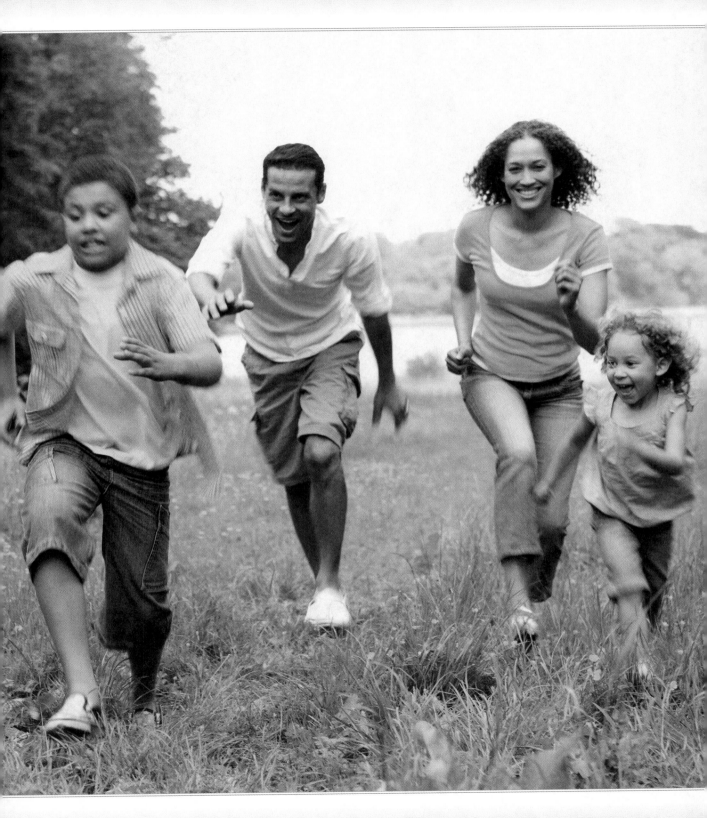

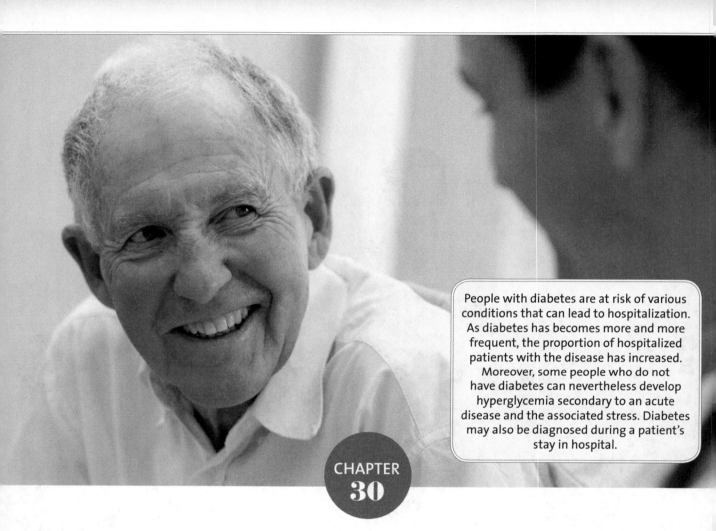

People with diabetes are at risk of various conditions that can lead to hospitalization. As diabetes has becomes more and more frequent, the proportion of hospitalized patients with the disease has increased. Moreover, some people who do not have diabetes can nevertheless develop hyperglycemia secondary to an acute disease and the associated stress. Diabetes may also be diagnosed during a patient's stay in hospital.

CHAPTER
30

People with Diabetes and Hospitalization

Why is hospitalization a relevant topic?

People with diabetes present various risks that predispose them to hospitalization. As diabetes has becomes more and more frequent, the proportion of hospitalized patients with the disease has increased. Moreover, some people who do not have diabetes can develop hyperglycemia secondary to an acute disease and the associated stress. Diabetes may also be diagnosed during a patient's stay in hospital.

Is it important to control blood glucose levels when staying in the hospital?

Blood glucose control is important while staying in the hospital because hyperglycemia can increase the risk of complications (e.g., infections) and lead to longer hospital stays. Hypoglycemia should also be avoided since it too is associated with a risk of complications.

What should blood glucose targets be while staying in the hospital?

Although the subject of optimal blood glucose targets has yet to be completely settled, it is generally recommended that a level between 5 and 8 mmol/L be maintained before meals and under 10 mmol/L at all times. Generally, targets for people in intensive care in the hospital are between 6 mmol/L and 10 mmol/L.

What is used to treat hyperglycemia and diabetes in the hospital?

Generally speaking, if the person's regular treatment is oral or injectable antidiabetics, it may be continued if the person is able to eat, has acceptable blood glucose levels, and has a stable clinical condition. However, in many situations, insulin is the medication of choice in the hospital. In fact, antidiabetic medications are sometimes contraindicated in acute cases (e.g., acute renal failure) or may not be given if the person is unable to eat or is required to fast before a procedure. Blood glucose may also rise significantly because of illness, stress, or certain types of medications (e.g., corticosteroids). In these cases, insulin must be used temporarily. It is delivered by subcutaneous injection or short-acting insulin is given intravenously.

How should a person with diabetes prepare for planned hospitalization?

People who are planning a stay in the hospital should inform the health care team that normally oversees their diabetes treatment and other health issues. Ideally, hospitalized patients provide a list of their medications, which they can obtain from their pharmacist. Vigilance is necessary, since hospitals often make mistakes about insulin. Be very precise about the type of insulin and the doses you take; simply saying that you take "short-acting" or "slow-acting" is not sufficient to determine the proper treatment. A record of your blood glucose readings and, if possible, your glycated hemoglobin levels is also useful.

If you use the insulin pump, you are strongly advised to discuss an action plan with your endocrinologist before checking into the hospital. The health care team should be informed that you use a pump. If your condition allows it, you can manage your own treatment while in the hospital, provided you are authorized to do so by your attending physician. If you do so, inform your health care team about your blood glucose levels and any modifications to your insulin doses.

Do insulin needs change during hospitalization?

Insulin needs can vary greatly during a stay in the hospital. As explained above, they can increase because of the illness, the associated stress, or certain medications. In other situations, they may decrease, for example if nutrition intake varies greatly from what is normally eaten at home. If any changes were made to your usual treatment, be sure you understand them before you check out of the hospital. It is also important to see your doctor soon after your stay to ensure that your medications are properly adjusted.

Are there any precautions that should be taken when going to the hospital for outpatient surgery?

Some types of surgery or procedures can be done in a single day and do not require hospitalization. People taking antidiabetic medications or insulin should take some precautions, however. A procedure that requires you to fast beforehand generally requires skipping the dose of antidiabetics and rapid- or short-acting insulin and, in some cases, reducing the intermediate- or long-acting insulin dose. Be sure that you have clear instructions regarding your diabetes or any other health condition before the day of your procedure.

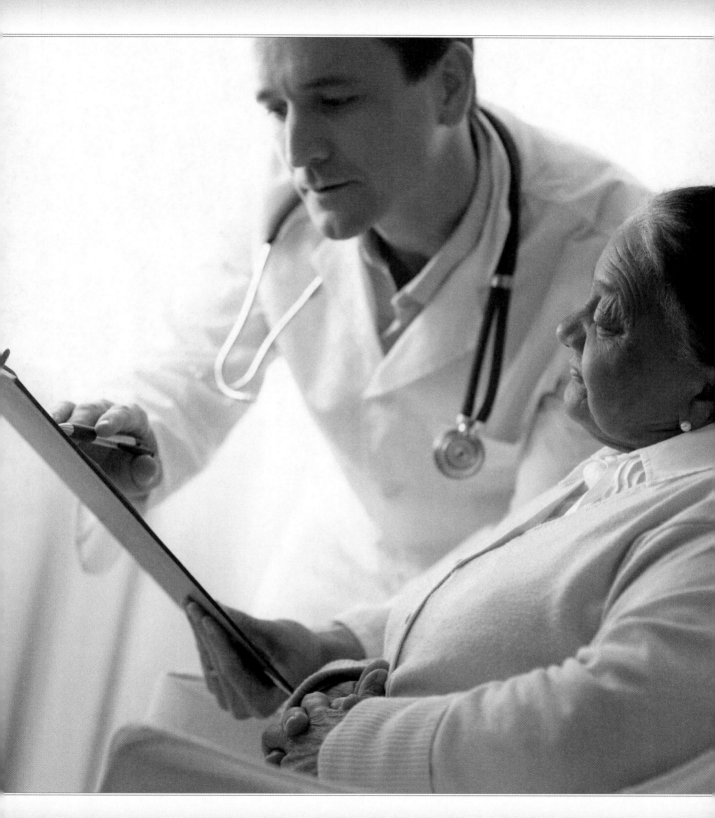

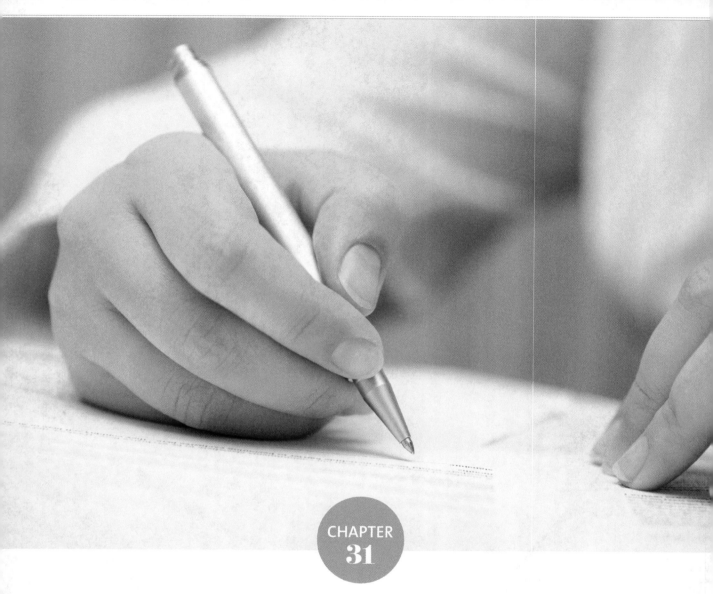

Diabetes
Follow-up Tools

How is diabetes "managed"?

Managing diabetes presents a number of challenges. Medical follow-ups, blood glucose self-monitoring, diet, exercise and medication are all important aspects of treatment that people with diabetes have to keep in mind at all times.

It can all seem overwhelming. Diabetes forces people to reconsider their entire lifestyle and make a long-term commitment to managing the condition. The easiest way to improve treatment is to take things one step at a time instead of trying to change every habit at once. People should set clear and realistic goals, congratulate themselves for each goal successfully achieved, and learn from any difficulties they encounter.

Are there any tools to help with diabetes follow-up?

People with diabetes have several tools available to help them follow up on their disease. A self-monitoring logbook is obviously essential. Another useful tool is a journal of personal goals, listing objectives relating to five important aspects of the follow-up: medical follow-up, care, diet, medication and well-being. People are advised to select any number of these objectives and rank them in order of priority (for example, from 1 to 5).

It is a good idea to consult this journal from time to time. Checking it periodically can help keep track of progress, understand why some goals are more difficult to reach than others, figure out how to reach them, or set new objectives. (*See the model journal on pages 310 to 313.*)

Is there a tool to help manage diet?

A meal plan drawn up with the aid of a dietitian is an essential tool for people with diabetes.

Which tests and targets help achieve optimal control of diabetes?

Medical follow-up of a person with diabetes includes various tests, including tests for blood glucose, glycated hemoglobin (A1C), blood lipids and blood pressure. Remember that glycated hemoglobin is used to determine how the blood sugar has been controlled over the last three months.

Target values for the various tests or measurements are presented in the "Targets for optimal control" chart on page 314.

How are the test results used?

Test results give doctors the tools to choose the appropriate treatment for a person with diabetes, to assess its effectiveness, and to make the necessary adjustments. The test follow-up journal (*see page 315*) can be used to keep track of relevant information, including test results. These results let a person with diabetes track treatment as it evolves and discuss it with the doctor. They can even be used as motivational tools.

JOURNAL OF PERSONAL GOALS

The following is a list of goals for people with diabetes. Choose the ones that are most important to you (a maximum of 5) and number them according to their priority. Periodically revise the objectives you choose today.

Dates					
MEDICAL FOLLOW-UP					
See the doctor at least twice a year					
Stay informed about the results of tests and examinations					
Get blood pressure checked					
Check microalbuminuria once a year					
See the ophthalmologist regularly, according to recommendations					

	Dates					
CARE AND RECOMMENDATIONS						
Record blood glucose levels in self-monitoring logbook and analyze them as recommended						
Check blood glucose more often when ill						
Compare readings from the blood glucose meter with a blood test at least once a year						
Have carbohydrates on hand at all times (at least two portions of 15 g each)						
Inspect my feet every day						
Do not smoke						
Exercise regularly (every day if possible)						
Wear a diabetic ID bracelet or pendant						
Inform driving authorities — in Quebec, the Société d'assurance automobile du Québec (SAAQ)						

	Dates					
DIET						
Eat the recommended amount of carbohydrates at every meal						
Eat balanced meals (carbohydrates, proteins, fats)						
Choose food rich in fiber						
Have the recommended snack in the evening						
Eat at regular hours						
Measure my food portions from time to time						
Keep a regular food journal						
Eat only recommended fats						
Drink alcohol only with food						

	Dates					
MEDICATION						
Take medications as prescribed by the doctor						
Know the name of my antidiabetic medications						
In my self-monitoring logbook, write the name of my diabetes medications and any changes in dosage						
Keep an updated list of all medications (doses and frequency) and bring it to all medical appointments						
Apply insulin dose adjustment rules						
Know the best times to take medications						
Know how to manage a skipped dose of antidiabetic medications						
Make sure that over-the-counter drugs or natural products will not worsen my diabetes						

	Dates					
WELL-BEING						
Identify stress factors that affect me the most						
Improve my reactions to stress						
Set aside at least 10 minutes a day for relaxation						
Speak to my support network about my diabetes						
Manage my time in a way that meets my needs						

	Dates					
MY PERSONAL GOALS						

Signature : _____

TARGETS FOR OPTIMAL CONTROL

Glucose

Glycated hemoglobin (A1C)	≤ 7% (for most)
Fasting or before-meal blood glucose	4 mmol/L – 7 mmol/L
Blood glucose 2 hours after a meal	5 mmol/L – 10 mmol/L (Tailor to individual: if possible 5 mmol/L – 8 mmol/L if A1C > 7%)

Lipid profile

LDL cholesterol	≤ 2,0 mmol/L (or decrease by ≥ 50%)

Kidneys

Albumin/creatinine ratio	< 2.0 mg/mmol
Albuminuria	< 20 µg/min or < 30 mg/day

Other

Blood pressure	< 130/80 mm Hg
Normal weight	65 years old : BMI* 18.5 – 24.9**
Waist measurement	M : < 102 cm (40 inches) W : < 88 cm (35 inches)

* BMI = body mass index (weight in kg/height in m^2)
** For people over the age of 65, normal BMI can range from slightly above 18.5 to a value located in the overweight range (BMI 25.0 to 29.9), according to the Canadian Guidelines for Body Weight Classification in Adults.
***These values apply to black or white people. For Asians, the measurements are < 90 for men and < 80 for women.

Name : _____

TEST FOLLOW-UP JOURNAL

Date								
Weight (kg)								
Height (m)								
BMI (kg/m2)								
Waist measurement (cm)								
Blood pressure (< 130/80 mm Hg)								
Blood glucose (blood test): • Before meal: 4 mmol/L – 7 mmol/L								
• After meal: 5 mmol/L – 10 mmol/L (Tailor to individual: 5 mmol/L – 8 mmol/L if A1C > 7 %)								
Glycated hemoglobin (A1C) ($\leq$ 7 % for most)								
LDL cholesterol ($\leq$ 2,0 mmol/L)								
Albumin/creatinine ratio (< 2.0 mg/mmol)								
Albuminuria (< 20 µg/min or < 30 mg/day)								
Creatinine clearance (Normal $\geq$ 1,5 ml/s/1.73 m² or 90 ml/min/1.73 m²)								

Annexe

BLOOD GLUCOSE CONVERSION CHART

mmol/L*	mg/dL**	mmol/L	mg/dL
1.4	25	11.2	202
1.6	29	11.6	209
1.8	32	12.0	216
2.0	36	12.4	223
2.4	43	12.8	230
2.8	50	13.2	238
3.2	58	13.6	245
3.6	65	14.0	252
4.0	72	14.4	259
4.4	79	14.8	266
4.8	86	15.2	274
5.2	94	15.6	281
5.6	101	16.0	288
6.0	108	16.4	295
6.4	115	16.8	302
6.8	122	17.2	309
7.0	126	17.6	317
7.2	130	18.0	324
7.6	137	18.5	333
8.0	144	19.0	342
8.4	151	19.5	351
8.8	158	20.0	360
9.2	166	20.5	369
9.6	173	21.0	378
10.0	180	21.5	387
10.4	187	22.0	396
10.8	194	22.5	405

Target values before meals and at bedtime

* mmol/L x 18 = mg/dL   ** mg/dL ÷ 18 = mmol/L